IN AND OUT

*My life as a guest of the NHS
for its fifty years and five,
as both an in- and out-patient*

Ray Hill

The Book Guild Ltd
Sussex, England

First published in Great Britain in 2001 by
The Book Guild Ltd
25 High Street
Lewes, East Sussex
BN7 2LU

Typesetting in Times by
SetSystems Ltd, Saffron Walden, Essex

Printed in Great Britain by
Antony Rowe Ltd, Chippenham, Wiltshire

A catalogue record for this book is
available from the British Library

ISBN 1 85776 559 1

*This book is dedicated to
my wife Irene, and the NHS.
Without the love of one
and the care of both, I would not
have been able to write this book.*

I could easily have been my own 'ghost' writer.
30 September 1998

ACKNOWLEDGEMENTS

With grateful thanks to all concerned, from the surgeons, doctors, nursing staff and physiotherapists, to the 'bottle washers' and 'bedpan carriers'.

Thanks to Glenice and Al (Dr Glenice Heaton and Dr Ali Ahmed), for their generosity and their friendship and to Irene's niece, Susan, for her work on the manuscript.

Also thanks to my son, David, my friends, Joan and Eric, Elsie and Bill, Pauline and Leslie, for always being there for me.

FOREWORD

This book has been written as a tribute to that much maligned group of people who are known collectively as the National Health Service.

The consultants, doctors, nurses, physiotherapists, radiographers and every other person that gathered together in their respective hospitals, are, or should be the pride of our country, irrespective of colour or creed, and not forgetting our general practitioners in their group practices throughout the land.

When you read this book you will find that there have been hiccups along the way but in spite of those I believe that we have the best hospitals in the world.

Successive governments over the years have not helped them maintain the high standards we expect from hospitals due to serious under-funding.

This no more evident since the end of this book, than the years of the lottery and its billions of pounds spread far and wide. Plus the fiasco of all fiascos 'the Dome'.

R. Hill
November 2000

1

My birth would seem the best place to start this story, 20 June 1928. For that occasion was my first introduction to the 'hospital' way of life. It seems that I had been giving my mother a very unhappy and trying time prior to my arrival on this worldly scene. Then I finally blotted my copybook. Apparently I kicked, struggled, fought and cried so much, that my mother decided then and there that I was to be the last of the line, at least as far as she herself was concerned. For just one like me was enough. This she vehemently declared.

So it all began.

A long period of time elapsed before my next hospital visit. Fifteen years to be exact. For my own GP, a big Irishman, had always been the one to patch up my bloody nose, bloody knees, and all the other minor cuts and bruises. Then, at last, came the something even he couldn't fix for me.

Agonising pains in my right side, together with bouts of nausea, had at last forced me to call at the surgery. I sat there cold and damp, after having trudged through drizzling rain. I felt really sorry for myself, and my surroundings didn't make me feel any better. The surgery was a drab, cold and miserable room, warmed only by a small gas fire that spluttered and popped alarmingly, and seemed destined to give out at any minute. Some of the other occupants of the room seemed about to do the same, as they also coughed and wheezed, and muttered 'Oh dears' from behind overworked and sodden handkerchiefs. A round-shouldered and sorry group we must have looked. The only sign of life and vitality from any of us was when the doctor's bell rang for the next patient. Then the air was charged with tension, as we all tried to remember who we followed in our turn, and to check that no one was queue jumping.

Eventually, it was my turn, and into the doctor's room I shuffled, a very frightened and trembling kid.

'My God Raymond, you look frightful,' he boomed. 'Sit down and tell me what ails you.'

I lowered myself wearily into the chair with a groan, and mumbled, 'I feel very sick and I have a pain in my side.' He lifted his bulk easily out of his chair and came round to examine me. Gently, he eased me out of my seat and practically carried me over to the couch. As I lay back and closed my eyes, I heard the sound of running water, then a brusque order in Manchester-Irish.

'Swallow these tablets for me, and you will soon feel much better.' I strongly doubted it, but did as I was instructed and washed the tablets down with the water provided. After a very brief examination, the doctor went back and sat down at his desk and started to write.

'Well Raymond, if you were a girl I would say you were pregnant, but as you are not, I will send you to the hospital for a check up, for your symptoms seem to point to a "grumbling" appendix.'

Bloody hell, I thought to myself, if this appendix is only grumbling, I really hope that it doesn't decide to be angry on me.

So, the following morning, armed with my doctor's letter of introduction, I made my way to our largest City Hospital. To a scared kid of fifteen, it looked a forbidding and mammoth place, there seemed to be people everywhere, and even the streets seemed to be crowded with nurses. After tentative enquiries at the lodge, I made my way nervously through the gates and into, for the second time, a hospital. Well immediately, my second visit was almost my last, for unseen by me, a large plum-coloured ambulance flew round the corner, arriving with a group of people from various parts of the city. It took a mighty leap on my part to prevent that vehicle of mercy with its out-patients from making me an extremely quick in-patient. As I scuttled away, the driver's Mancunian tongue lashed me mercilessly, so that my face turned the same colour as his ambulance.

What could happen to me next, I wondered, as I made my way into the great hall where there seemed to be hundreds of people, some strolling about, but the majority just sat in rows on hard forms. Whether sitting or walking, the main thing in common seemed, to my eyes, to be rather sad looking faces and nobody seemed to talk to each other.

'Well here I am, what do I do now?' I asked myself. I gazed furtively about, and there behind a window marked 'Appointments' sat a large and wholesome lady with a beaming smile. She beckoned me over and took from me my now very crumpled letter. I sat by the window while she filled in my name, address, date of birth etc. on some form or other. As I waited, I felt slightly more at ease, but then this feeling was shattered as the lady told me to find a seat and wait for my name to be called. Find a seat indeed. Where, in that crowd, was I going to find a seat, me and my ever 'grumbling' and painful appendix?

Then, at last, after vain meanderings up and down those rows of seats, I spotted a place, if you could possibly call it that. I dashed quickly forward to perch my left cheek precariously on about six inches of wooden form, next to what seemed to be a mountain of a man, with a beard almost as big as his belly.

So began the long vigil, and as the hours slowly passed, this sad youth was steadily reaching a rather dejected and frantic state, with my appendix hurting like blazes on my right side, and this huge scowling hulk of a man, glowering down on me on my left. We both sat and watched people slowly follow each other in a steady, if somewhat drawn out, procession through a door guarded by a smiling grey-haired lady, my first true sight of a National Health Service 'Angel of Mercy', a nurse. As she called out names, she seemed to have a kind word for everyone, old and young alike.

Then suddenly, at the sound of a name, instantly and without any warning, the big man stood up. He went up, but I went down, and down with a resounding bang! Flat on the floor! With the combination of my pain, and hurt to my youthful ego, my tears began to flow freely. This brought to my side and aid, the nurse from the door. She reached me in a flash and to my utter amazement, she was also crying, with tears rolling down her cheeks uncontrollably. Her tears though, were not of sorrow, but of riotous laughter for, as she quickly explained and described, the huge man's rise and my subsequent fall, had been, from her own, and as she pointed out, all the many other laughing faces, all other points of view, highly amusing. As I sat there on the floor, I looked carefully at the people nearby and noticed the difference in their faces and eyes. Yes, eyes that had been sad were now twinkling gaily, and faces that had been creased with pain and anxiety were now momentarily wreathed in smiles, and believe it or not, they were now even talking to each other. In those fleeting seconds, as my teenage mind took in this scene, I realised that I must always try to laugh at myself in adversity and pain. For not only did I think it might help me, but more importantly, it might help the others around me.

In a flash that thought flew from my mind, and back came the throbbing pain. Soon though, my name was called, and then it was my turn to enter a Surgeon's domain for the first time. I wondered frighteningly what was going to happen to me. As it turned out, I was to have little chance to find out, for our meeting was all too brief.

On the direction of the nurse, I had slipped off my shoes and socks, and had wearily laid myself down on the bed. As I looked up to the ceiling, the room began to spin alarmingly, and my vision became very hazy. Then through the haze, a blurred figure appeared. 'Hello son, now what seems to be the trouble?' said a kindly voice.

'A terrible pain, sir, here in my side,' I replied weakly.

4

'Where?' he asked and, before I could reply, 'there?' And as he spoke, he jabbed his finger into my side. There appeared to be a blinding flash of light, and I passed into oblivion.

2

My eyes flickered open. Slap! Slap! Slap! I felt my face being gently slapped, what on earth was happening to me?

'Come on, spit it out, there's a good lad,' a seemingly distant voice was saying. More slaps, and again the request, 'Come on, there's a good lad, out with it.' Spit what out? Though very bemused, I was getting very mad. Suddenly I gave a gigantic heave, and out of my mouth flew an object, I know not what.

'Oh my God,' I moaned, and became violently sick.

I heaved and heaved, and heaved again.

'It's all over now boy, you will feel fine soon,' a gentle voice said to me.

'What is over? Where am I?' I begged. And then, once again, overpowering nausea. I became conscious of a dark round face, which seemed to be all flashing teeth and sparkling brown eyes.

'How is he nurse?'

'Sickly still.' This was another voice from the opposite side of the bed I had found myself in. As I turned my head to see the owner of this voice, I saw a tall elegant lady in a dark blue uniform, and on her head was a beautiful lace hat. She began to gently wipe my sweating forehead. I lay there, looking up at them both, a very mixed up and frightened kid.

'What has happened to me please?' I begged to know.

'Well Raymond, you have parted with your very trouble-some appendix,' she told me. I stared at her in disbelief until once again nausea overcame me, and as I retched and retched, both of these kind ladies kept on repeating

6

words to me, words that I was to hear often in the years ahead.

'Big deep breaths Raymond, and open your mouth and try to breathe deeply. Come on try very hard.' Try hard I did, but it in no way helped at all. For then, and in the years to come, whenever I felt sick after an operation, I was. And no amount of deep breathing exercises made the slightest difference.

I soon fell into a deep sleep and after what seemed a few short hours, awoke again happily to find that the sickness seemed to have left me, and also that the pain in my side was more bearable, if far from comfortable. Lifting my head slightly I took my first look around the inside of a hospital ward. My bed was first on the right as you entered the place, so that to my right, and all along the opposite wall, were some thirty beds or so. All of which seemed to be occupied. Another feature I quickly noticed was that even though it was still daylight, all the heavy dark blinds were partially drawn, and that all the windows were criss-crossed with broad white tape. When my coloured nurse came to check how I was doing, I asked her, why the white tape? She told me it was to stop them from splintering if a bomb fell nearby. Not a pleasant thought as I lay directly beneath one of these large windows.

As my eyes moved slowly along the beds they were, in turn, met with varied reactions. A half smile, a broad grin, a cheery wave, and in some cases, complete disregard. This last attitude was disconcerting to a young lad in the strangest surroundings of his short life. It was early yet for me to learn about patients, and their reaction to hospital life, and to other occupants of the ward.

Then all my attention was taken up by the bedlam and what to my ears were never ending cries of distress.

'Nurse!'

'Bottle please, nurse!'

'Nurse, bring me a bed-pan ... quickly!' This, a very frantic cry, a real demand for assistance. In answer to all these impassioned pleas, nurses and white-coated men and women were running and scurrying hither and thither, carrying an odd and strange assortment of glass and stainless steel receptacles.

The recipients of the glass bottles plunged them beneath the sheets and, in a few seconds, strained faces suddenly became relaxed, and looks of utter contentment shone through. Arms would stretch out holding their handiwork, some shyly, as a bare inch of fluid swished about in the bottom of the bottle, or others, who were proudly showing bottles filled almost to the brim with frothing liquid.

The bedpan routine was very different, a comparatively private affair, with the drawing of the curtains heralding the arrival of the bright shiny pan. The mixture of grunts and groans that came from the curtains soon afterwards, seemed rather frightening to my immature ears. It was later that I was to learn the agony and ecstasy of the bedpan ritual. Bedpan removal was usually a very quick affair, with one arm outstretched and the finger and thumb of the other hand firmly gripping the nose as the very unfortunate remover made a hasty dash for the sluice.

Taking up the central position in the ward was a large steaming container of I knew not what. It looked a real shining monster and my mind boggled at what it might contain. Before my eyes flashed the image of hooded Spanish Inquisitors bending over hot tools of torture. I shuddered and quickly turned away.

Night-time came, and with it the visitors. A steady stream of people bearing smiles and gifts, with the gifts in most cases being received more readily than the smiles or hand-shakes seemed to be. As my family had been to see me earlier while I was asleep, I was able to lie back and take note of the varied reactions between patients and the visitors.

There was the devoted wife with her neat parcel of cakes and sandwiches, forever smiling and making pleasant conversation. On the other hand, there was the overpowering and overbearing wife with her bouquet of flowers and ceaseless noisy chatter. Always on the move to be sure everyone could see her fussing over her poor unfortunate spouse, who was constantly having himself jerked from side to side, whilst the misguided lady straightened what was already a very comfortable bed. Then there were the relatives and friends of other patients, who sat there, straight-faced and staring, or with fixed smiles which they hoped, I was sure, would pass off as cheerful.

The noise of the visitor's arrival and the dragging of chairs to the bedside gradually subsided, and I was able to catch various snatches of conversation, just the odd word here and there. Two beds away a group of sad-faced people stood around the poor occupant and gazed down at him as though they were from the local undertakers and he was a prospective client.

'Hello, our Fred, you are looking better,' said one dead pan face, and then as he moved back to the end of the bed, he said in a whisper loud enough to be heard all around the ward, 'I don't think he will last much longer, but maybe it is all for the best.' To my amazement, everyone in the group seemed to nod in complete agreement. I just couldn't believe it was true.

Next to me though, it was a completely different story. This patient had had his operation just two days before, and apparently it had been rather a large one. Consequently he was barely able to move at all. His visitors, all male, had obviously arrived to cheer him up, come what may. The jokes were flowing fast and furious, and they were all convulsed with laughter. That is all except the poor patient, my immediate neighbour. For as I looked at him, I saw his hands grip his sheets tightly, so tightly that I could see his knuckles turn white with the pressure. His face was a picture of restrained and withheld laughter. It was only later that I was to learn that riotous laughter and stitches are not compatible. Fortunately for my companion, there was the sound of a bell ringing, and I saw all the people start to assemble their belongings, as well as dirty pyjamas etc. put away their chairs, and make for the door.

Departure itself was a sight to behold. There the ones who made an immediate dash for the exit and were gone. Others who meandered along slowly, smiling and nodding at everyone as they passed by. Lastly, there was the type who walked slowly backwards smiling and waving constantly to their loved ones, as they tried to add valuable seconds to the visiting hour.

The exodus over, I turned to face my neighbour, and in doing so I really felt, for the first time, my own stitches, and I must have shown it visibly.

'Take it easy son, try not to move about too much yet,' he advised kindly.

'Thanks, I will try not to,' I replied, then, 'That visiting seemed a bit hectic, you seemed to be in real agony.'

'Oh yes I was, but they all meant well and that is all that matters. For these are the times when you really find out who your friends are.'

After these profound words, he asked, 'Does it hurt much?'

'Yes it is beginning to,' I answered.

'Well you will feel better after a good night's sleep.' He seemed to know, but I doubted it very much.

'Sleep?' I queried, 'I am sure I won't be able to sleep here.'

'You will son, you will.' This he said in a very knowing voice. How can he be so sure I will sleep, I thought to myself, how could anyone with all the noise and activity that always seems to be going on? There seemed to be another sudden scurry of action as the bottles and bedpans were circulated again, neither of which I wanted. Then the ward seemed to suddenly quieten down and almost sound peaceful. Various nurses popped into the ward to shout a cheery 'Good night lads' then off they went.

Eventually Sister came in, accompanied by another nurse and white-coated orderly. They moved around the ward and stood for a few seconds at the end of each bed in quiet conversation. When they reached my bed, I heard Sister say, 'This is young Raymond, emergency appendectomy today. He still isn't sure what it's all about yet.' How right she was!

'Injection and a sleeping-pill tonight, it is all written up for him. And he hasn't passed any water yet.' I felt myself blush as three pairs of female eyes seemed to stare right through me. At last they moved on and out of the ward.

Minutes later, the orderly returned with a flourish, propelling a trolley laden with the goodnight drinks. 'Tea, coffee, Horlicks or Ovaltine, come on fellows, name your poison.' She had served everyone in no time at all. 'Now, young man, what can I do for you?' She laughed, 'Don't answer that. For one thing you are too young, and for another, you are too weak.' Her cheerfulness made me feel the best I had felt all day. My God! It seemed a long time since I first entered the hospital. Was it only this morning? It was almost too hard to believe.

Back to earth.

'I wouldn't mind a drink of tea please. Two sugars.'

'I will give you a feeder,' she said. I watched her pour the tea into what seemed to be a small teapot. What on earth is that thing, I thought, but I quickly realised the benefit of this useful object. As I was able to sip my tea through the spout without having to strain and disturb myself into a sitting position to do so. Ah, the wonders of science.

A few minutes later the nurse arrived carrying a small metal dish, in which I could see what to my eyes seemed to be a large needle. I must have gone white at thought of what was to come, for she smiled and said, 'Don't worry Raymond, you'll hardly feel a thing.' The orderly came along to help me roll over gently onto my side, and as I did, I realised for the first time, that I only had on some kind of night-shirt that somehow was loosely tied at the back. As I lay there, bare-bottomed for all to see, I didn't have time to feel embarrassed. For a quick slap, followed by a sharp prick, gave me a lot more to think about.

'Bloody hell,' I bellowed, and jerked away. This caused a lot more pain and consternation, for the sudden movement made me pull on the stitches in my side. Oh dear, I wasn't very happy at all.

After they had tucked me in tightly, adjusted my pillows,

and made me as comfortable as possible, I felt much better. Even though I still felt as tender as a lump of well-beaten steak, now both in my side and bottom. Before the nurse moved away she bent over and whispered gently some tiny words of advice.

'With injections Raymond, learn to relax and accept them. You will find this makes them much more bearable.' I wasn't to know it then, but those words were to save me such a lot of pain and discomfort in the years that lay ahead.

'Don't hesitate to call if you need me in the night, I will only be sat there, a few feet away from the end of your bed. Now try to use the bottle for me if you can, it's there on your locker.' She gingerly ruffled my hair and said a quiet 'Goodnight.' Soon I was asleep, with a very eventful day well and truly over.

3

My eyes flickered open. Something was wrong. What was it? Then I knew, it was the noise. Sheer bedlam, or so it seemed. It was like Piccadilly Bus Station in the rush hour. I looked at my watch. My God, it wasn't even six o'clock. The orderly was dashing round with clanging metal wash-bowls, banging them on locker tops and filling them with water, and accompanying the actions with cries of 'Wakey, wakey gentlemen. Come on, washtime is here. Be as quick as you can.' She certainly didn't intend for anyone to remain asleep for long, that was for sure.

I stretched my legs, and then tried to sit upright.

'Oh! Oh!' I moaned out loud, and flopped down on my back again.

'Well Raymond,' I said to myself, 'we are not going to try that again, not for a while anyway.'

'Tea Ray?' a cheery voice enquired. It was one of the walking wounded doing the early morning tea round, a noble and necessary duty in all hospitals.

'Yes please, gladly.' My mouth felt as rough as sandpaper. I had barely finished the nectar when the bowl clanging orderly arrived at my bedside. Before I realised what was happening, she was busily washing my hands and face.

'Steady on. I can wash myself you know.' I think I was more embarrassed than anything else. The thought of being washed by a woman in front of a ward full of men seemed to be a bit much.

'Shut up, lie back and enjoy it,' she ordered.

'Enjoy it, at this time of the morning, even the birds aren't up yet,' I snapped back.

13

'Yes they are, you can hear them singing through the kitchen window.'

'Manchester birds don't sing, they cough.' I was determined to have the last word.

'Now, now young man, don't be so cheeky. I have got to shave you yet.' As she gently threatened me, her face was covered in a big smile. I shut up immediately, for I had only just reached the shaving age, and as I wasn't too happy shaving myself, I certainly didn't relish the idea of antagonising the person who was going to have to do it for me.

Having made her point and won the battle, she gently stroked my cheeks and said, 'I think we can leave the shave today.' As she cleared away the washing utensils, she noticed my empty bottle.

'I see you haven't used your bottle yet. You must try harder. Drink as much as you can, it will help you.' Two minutes after she had left me I was asleep again.

I opened my eyes to a hive of industry. Nurses were dashing round, handing out trays containing cups and saucers etc., all in preparation for breakfast. Breakfast! Food! Oh the thought of it turned my stomach over. My nausea returned and I started to retch again. I spent the next ten minutes heaving, and staring into the bottom of a shiny metal basin, a position I was to occupy regularly in the future.

The Staff Nurse in charge of the breakfast detail wisely gave me a miss, and for the sake of the other lads, quickly had me encircled with the curtains. After half an hour or so I felt a little better, and once the first meal of the day was over, my drapes were pulled back once more.

My bout of sickness had really unsettled me, so I lay there as still as could be, frightened to move and very unhappy. To keep my mind off my pain and sickness, I started to really take notice of the activity and work that was being carried out in the ward. One nurse was touring the place with the 'bedpan' and 'bottle' trolley, a ritual after meals that I was to get used to in the years ahead. Though

14

as for myself, I could never educate my bladder and bowels to work in co-ordination with the medical timetable. Another nurse was busily going round taking temperature and pulse, just to keep a close check on all our conditions, the thermometer being a very good guide as to whether you were a 'goer' or a 'stayer'. The rest of the staff were on bed detail, working in pairs. As I watched the way they rolled the occupants of the beds from side to side, and then finally, the big heave, as they dragged the victim up the bed to his resting place on his freshly shaken and soft pillows, I thought to myself, I hope they don't do that to me when it is my turn. I will die, I am sure I will.

My thoughts were interrupted by the arrival of the day Sister, plus another needle. As she rolled down the clothes, I remembered the advice I had been given after my last injection. So I turned away and gritted my teeth.

'Relax, Raymond relax,' she advised me gently. Not me. Oh no not me. I just continued to lie there all tense and tight. Wham! It was as though I had been hit by a battering ram.

'Oh, Oh, Oh!' I turned my head and looked at the Sister with tears in my eyes. 'That really hurt. Did you have to stick it in so hard?' It was still all very new to me and I was easily upset.

'I told you to relax. You should try to, it will make things so much easier for you.' She was trying to be helpful. As she was talking she was rubbing her hand over the spot on my backside where she had done the damage. Now that part of it I did like!

'You haven't used your bottle yet, I see.' Her words quickly brought me back to earth.

'No, not yet. I don't feel the need to.' I thought to myself, 'They are all obsessed with this bottle lark!'

'Well you must keep trying to, and drink plenty of fluids,' and off she went.

By this time the bed-makers had arrived, both for my neighbour and myself. As they pulled the curtains around each of us, I promised myself that if he didn't cry out, I wouldn't. One of the nurses I had was a big pleasant coloured girl.

'Hello there, boy, remember me? I was the one who brought you from theatre yesterday,' her voice seemed to sing. I nodded and half-smiled, but I was terrified. If she starts to throw me about like the others, she will burst my stitches for sure. Brother, I had a lot to learn.

They rolled down the clothes, leaving me exposed, except for just my little tied-at-the-back nightie. To my horror, they rolled me over, ever so easily, undid the ties and whipped it off. I was shattered. There I lay for them both to see, wearing only the dressing that covered my operation. To add to my embarrassment was the sight of my stomach and 'privates', bare of hair. All had gone. My white face turned bright red, and that colour I am sure, slowly spread down to my toes. I didn't know whether to cover my eyes or my 'privates' with my hands. In the end I decided just to close my eyes and do nothing. From my locker, the nurses took a pair of pyjamas and quickly slipped them on. As they tied the cord carefully over my middle, the happy coloured girl tickled my navel and said, 'Don't be shy love, you will soon get used to us.' They changed my sheets and made my bed, and finally came to the part I was dreading. Each one placed an arm under my armpit, ordered me to rest my chin on my chest, and then heaved me up the bed. To my amazement, I hardly felt a thing! They were great. Then they spoilt the whole thing. Yes, it was the empty urine bottle! Almost in unison, they both said, 'Haven't you used this yet? Come on you must try.' To my horror, they passed it to me, and told me to try there and then. One whistled and the other poured water from a large jug into a bowl. But all to no avail.

'Leave it there, and keep at it.' With that they pulled back the curtains and left. As I lay there nursing the bottle and trying to will myself to pass water, I felt as if every eye in the ward was on me.

The day passed quickly by, with me doing a fair amount of sleeping, and when I wasn't doing that, I spent most of

16

my time looking at my reflection in the bottom of a stainless steel vomiting dish. One thing I didn't do was eat. Even if I didn't eat, everyone seemed to be intent on one thing, and that was to stretch my poor bladder to bursting proportions. It seemed to be the aim of all and sundry, doctors, nurses and orderlies, to keep filling my water jug.

The day staff took their leave, to be replaced by the equally vigilant night nurses. By this time I was feeling most uncomfortable, my side was painful and I was very sickly. But the most disconcerting thing was my very swollen bladder. Every time I moved you could almost hear the water swishing about inside. Yet still they persisted in pouring fluids into me. It was only when I complained bitterly to the Night Sister 'If you want me to drink so much, why don't you pour it in through a tube', that her reply of 'If you don't hurry up and wee that is exactly what we have to do to get it out. And the tube will have to go up your penis', really shattered me.

'You're kidding me Sister, they don't do that.' Then in a voice that was almost a wail, 'Do they?' My answer to her nod was to reach for the accursed bottle and shove it quickly beneath my bedclothes and try again. I tried that hard that I became soaked in perspiration. It seemed that this was the only way any fluids were to escape from my body. Terrified now, I just lay there ignoring everything and everyone, and just willing myself to pass water. All other things were incidental. Another injection, my bed being straightened for the night, nothing else mattered but the thought, 'I must pass water, I must.'

The lights went out but I still lay there wide-awake and very worried. Eventually I must have dropped off, but been very restless, for I opened my eyes to see the nurse and the Night Sister beside my bed. Even as I opened my eyes, they were drawing the curtains around me. I was sweating pints and felt dreadful. I didn't even care when Sister rolled down my bedclothes, undid my pyjamas and placed my penis in a bottle and said, 'Come on Raymond, try really hard, and don't be shy.' Shy? I couldn't have cared if the Matron and the rest of the nurses in the hospital were stood around my bed. All I wanted to do now was wee. I stared at the ceiling, please God help me! Eventually the Sister gave up the 'bottle' way.

'Nurse, go and get me a bedpan,' she said.

'I don't want a bedpan Sister,' I begged, 'Honest I don't.' All my argument was to no avail. The pan arrived, and with it more help. So there was now the Sister, nurse and the orderly. They slid off my trousers, and with the Sister at one side of the bed and the nurse at the other, they started to ease me up into a sitting position, with the orderly behind me waiting with the bedpan. I had only had a minor operation, but as I reached an upright position, I felt as if I was being disembowelled. They lifted me gently and slid the pan under my bottom. Not more than a few seconds was I there, when whoosh! Water. Everywhere there was water. In the pan, in the bed, overflowing onto the floor, and even the girls were wet through. They didn't care. I didn't care. I sat there perched precariously on my stainless steel throne, supported by those lovely 'angels of mercy'. I was woefully weak. I was soaking wet. I was trouserless. Above all I was relieved and very happy. All three of them eased me carefully off the overflowing bedpan and gently back into a horizontal position. They quickly dressed me in clean pyjamas, changed my bed completely, sprinkled me liberally with talcum powder, and then left me. I could have kissed all three of them.

Sleep came, and it was long and restful. I awoke the next morning feeling great. The next few days passed quickly, with only one other occasion to cause me any concern. Again, it was in the middle of the night, nature was calling, and I was in dire need of a bedpan. I had put off the deed for as long as I could, hoping against hope that I would last out until I was able to get out of bed and go off under my own steam. It was not to be. 'Nurse,' I whispered to the girl who was sat at a table a few feet from the end of my bed. She was busily knitting. Though how she could see in that very subdued lighting I don't know.

'Bloody hell!' It was a stifled expletive, from which I gathered she had dropped a stitch.

'Sorry nurse, but I do need a bedpan.'

'You can't have one.'

'Please,' I begged, 'I am desperate.'

'Oh all right then.' Then off she trotted to the sluice. A few more minutes and she was back.

'I am not drawing the curtains. You can just sit there where I can see you.' She placed her arm under mine and eased me up, while she slid the pan under my behind. Wowee! My eyes popped out as I looked at her. She held her hand tightly over her mouth to prevent herself laughing out loud. For as the tender spots on my bottom knew, she had run the damn thing under the hot water tap. It was no wonder my eyes watered. I sat perched upright on my hard seat like some imitation 'Ghandi' surveying his followers. My audience, thankfully almost all being asleep, the one exception being my night nurse, who just sat looking at me.

'Well come on, get on with it,' she told me.

'I can't. Not with you sat staring at me. What do you think I am, a peep show?'

'You didn't seem to care the other night, the night of the great floods.'

'That was different then.'

'Yes I know it was, but hurry up because I want to carry on with my knitting.' Then she relented. 'Carry on then and I will go and brew up.' No sooner had she disappeared from sight when once more nature erupted. Phew! The smell was foul. I was thankful it was the dead of night, and not in the middle of the day. My life would have been unbearable. The nurse and orderly returned together, bringing with them the tea. As soon as they entered the ward they stopped dead in their tracks.

'Raymond, you are rotten!' I was back to teenage shyness again.

'I am so sorry but how do you think I feel.' They approached cautiously.

19

'Have you finished? If you haven't, hurry up or you will finish us.' I nodded.

'Come on then, let us clean you up, you smell like a sewage farm. It is a good job the others are all asleep or they would make us wheel you into Whitworth Park!' They did a marvellous job. They wiped me, washed me, powdered me, and then stripped and remade my bed again. Even to my young mind it was incredible how hospitals could get women and girls to do such work. I personally wouldn't be a nurse for a gold clock. My drink of tea disposed of, I settled down for the rest of the night, and I left them to carry on with the knitting.

Time slid easily by, and nothing more eventful happened, that is, until the morning of the tenth day. We had, as usual, had the beds made, plus a cursory visit by the Surgeon and his followers. So all was set for a quiet day. I casually watched Sister approach the steaming steriliser with her trolley, and watched her remove a few steaming articles. 'Someone is for it,' I thought, half-smilingly to myself. I didn't smile for long, for it was my bed she made for. As she drew the curtains about us, she said, 'Stitches out today my lad.' I must have paled visibly, for I didn't know what to expect.

'Will it hurt?' I asked tentatively.

'Not a bit,' she assured me. Then as I unfastened my pyjamas I lay back, firmly gripped the sides of my bed, closed my eyes and waited with baited breath. There came a sudden sharp pain as she expertly removed my small plaster dressing with a flourish.

'Ow!' I yelped.

'Sorry,' in a gentle voice.

'A really cold feeling now. Ice cold.' This, as she applied the spirit to clean and soften the stitches.

'O-O-Oh!' I jumped at the shock.

'Now here we go.' I still kept my eyes tightly closed. I would have liked to look but I was too much of a coward. Snip, snip, snip went the scissors and still no pain, so I boldly ventured the opening of one eye to see, to my amazement, a new dressing being taped over my scar. Then as she displayed them for me to see, ten black stitches on a gauze pad. I smiled for the first time since she had arrived at my bed.

'It didn't hurt a bit.' My voice now of the bravado of youth. As the curtains were pulled back I felt as if the entire ward were proud of this heroic young lad. Oh dear me, I had such a lot to learn.

The next day I waited eagerly for the ward round, for after it, I had been told I would be allowed up for the first time in ten days. I just couldn't wait. A ward round is indeed a sight to behold, with neat and tidy beds, no smoking, and definitely no talking. Nurses and patients alike, all awaiting the arrival of the entourage. Patients nervously waiting to see if all is going well or otherwise, and nurses terrified in case the Surgeon may suddenly ask them a question about a patient or complaint that they can't answer. The only person not concerned, but was going serenely about her tasks, was Sister. A babble of voices and here they are. The Surgeon, his secretary, House Doctors and, as this is a teaching hospital, a host of students. They all now trail behind Sister with the good lady reminding the Consultant what he cut off whom and when. My turn arrived in due course. A quick look at the scar, a big smile, and a few reassuring words. 'Up today young fellow, and home for the weekend.' As he was about to move out of the ward, he looked back and left with these words, 'By the way, don't make a habit of this sort of thing.' A quick wave and he was gone. How little we both knew about the future.

The excitement over, the daily routine began for all once again. As I lay there waiting impatiently for someone to help me get out of bed, the idea began to seep through that I could see to myself. For the urge to make for the toilet was becoming very strong, and anyway that is the first place every patient heads for at the earliest moment. That is as soon as he is mobile. I shouted across to the nurses clearing away the x-rays and medical notes from the ward round, 'Is it okay if I get up now?'

21

'No, definitely not. Wait until one of us comes to you.'

'Go away with you, I feel great.' With that I swung my legs out of the bed and stood up. Stood up that is, for about thirty seconds! For as my legs took my weight I promptly collapsed, and slowly disappeared under the bed. In answer to the warning shouts of the other patients, two nurses dashed across, and pulled me rather unceremoniously from under the bed. They half-carried, half-dragged me, to an armchair in the middle of the ward. There they both proceeded to give me a lecture on my wasting the time of everyone who had looked after me during my stay in hospital. I sat and listened with head bowed, and wishing that I had a hole to go and crawl into. Then I heard laughter, and looked around to see most of my fellow patients doubled up with laughter. Then, as I looked up at my two lecturers, I saw that they too were having great difficulty in keeping from laughing out loud. So once again my demise, my fall from glory, had helped to bring amusement to others around me. If I could, in any way provide that important commodity, laughter whilst in hospital, it could only do good. So let them laugh, I don't care!

The two nurses were about to move away after having put me in my place. 'Excuse me ladies.' They both turned towards me. 'Can you take me to the toilet please? And hurry or we will be too late.' I smiled as if to appease them.

'You little bugger, you,' they gasped. In a flash they lifted me up and we scurried up the ward to the sluice. One held the door back while the other one loosened the cord on my trousers. As they fell to the floor, I was plonked onto the seat and told to stay there until they returned for me. After all the trouble I had caused, I wouldn't have dared to go against their wishes, so I sat there patiently. I didn't mind though, for after a bedpan, a toilet seat is luxury indeed. To be able to relax, and sit in peace with nature is absolute and sheer bliss.

My remaining days were soon gone and I took my leave of all and sundry, and departed for home in an ambulance. My very first ride in one. Would it be my last?

22

4

Three years later, as a young National Serviceman in Germany, I presented myself before my unit's Medical Officer.

'Good morning Sir.'

'Well Corporal, what brought you here?' he asked. I was dying to tell him my legs, but thought better of it.

'A lump in my right groin Sir. It came after last week's football game.' He didn't move from his chair.

'Take your trousers down and move round here to me.' If he thought I was going to drop them, then shuffle across the floor to him, he was wrong. So I moved round his desk, faced him and then dropped them! He didn't have to move his eyes in any way at all, there was the lump, and everything else staring him in the face. He soon removed the smirk from mine. He grabbed hold of me.

'Cough,' he barked. I did, and nearly fainted. 'You have a hernia my man. A rupture.' He was now genuinely concerned. He picked up the phone. 'I am sending you to hospital right away.'

My feet never touched the floor after that. I was whisked outside into an ambulance, and away I went to the nearest military hospital. The MO had done his job well, for everyone was waiting for me. I was quickly examined again by a Major who confirmed the urgency. He looked at his watch. 'Have him ready in two hours.' Then off he went. I looked at the Sergeant who was in the room with us.

'That was quick, why all the rush?' I didn't want to sound scared, but I was.

'You will be fine, but you do have a bit of a bad tear,' he

23

said, 'so the sooner it is done the better. Now then, hop on this trolley and I will take you up to the ward.' Here we go again.

This was only a minor hospital, not one of the large military establishments, so consequently the trolley didn't have far to go. We soon entered a small ward. It contained, in my hurried glance, only a few beds. The main feature was that the largest wall was all glass, and meant that there was a lovely view of the surrounding countryside. Apparently, this was a newish wing built onto a small German hospital. The Sergeant helped me from the trolley to the bed. We were then joined by a very pretty female nurse. She surrounded the bed with screens, then commenced to help me undress.

'I have nothing with me. No pyjamas, towels or shaving things. You see, I didn't realise that events were going to move so rapidly.'

'Don't worry, I can fix you up with everything you are likely to need. Everything!' This she said whilst she was kneeling and removing my boots and gaiters. I looked down at her with a knowing glance over the top of my glasses.

'No, not that! And with your complaint you would be committing suicide.' By the time we had got down to the underwear, the Sergeant had returned, now wearing a white coat and carrying a tray. On it I could see hot water, a lather brush and an open razor. This is carrying military discipline a bit far I thought, I have already had one shave today.

'Off with your vest and pants Corp., I am going to shave you. No, not your chin, there.' He waved the razor towards the top of my legs. By this time I was lying there in my birthday suit. 'Well let's face it, as it is they couldn't even find your hernia, let alone operate on it.'

The nurse had been putting my things away in the locker. As she stood up and looked at me, then the Sergeant, she said, 'I think you will need a lawnmower, not a razor.' Then, laughingly skipped away, 'Talk about a walk in the Black Forest!'

24

I rolled over to let the Sergeant slip a towel under my stern and legs. He then started to lather busily away until he had covered all my pubic hairs thoroughly. That part I didn't mind at all, and the white foam stretched from my navel, down past my crutch, to just above my knees. My face must have registered the trepidation I was feeling, for he casually waved the razor across my right groin, roughly from about my hipbone down to my b—s! The edge of the blade was that near I cringed.

'That is where they will cut, not from up here, don't worry.' Don't worry he says, and he's waving the open razor about like 'Jack the Ripper'. He must be bloody joking! Worried? Oh no, I wasn't worried, I was sodding-well terrified. A quick dip of the razor in the mug of hot water, and he bent over me. With long smooth strokes he swept the blade across and down my stomach.

'Appendix out I see,' he pointed at my scar, 'neat, very neat.' Soon my middle was completely hair free. His attention was then concentrated on my thighs. Again the long smooth strokes, first on one leg and then the next. And still, happily no sign of blood. I allowed myself a half-smile.

'Why the smile Corporal?' my shaver asked.

'I was just thinking, two fierce false cuts and I could be arsing about for the rest of my life!'

He lifted each leg in turn, and lathered and shaved away until they were as smooth as a baby's bottom. 'Now for the crunch,' he said with a leer. A fresh lathering completed on my pride and joy, and he was ready for the tricky bit. I looked at myself, all lily-white and clean – except for one lump of fluffy white soap lather. Somewhere in there was 'me', well at least the part of me that seemed the most important at the time.

'I daren't look.'

'Well just lie back, close your eyes and pray.' This wasn't him; it was the nurse who returned armed with another tray. My eyes were shut tight, but I felt the blade gently moving over me.

'Ow!' I yelped, and prayed harder.

25

'Sorry, just a nick.' I felt my penis being lifted and stretched then lathered again. I didn't know which one of them was holding it, in this instance I didn't care either. More firm but gentle strokes and then it was over. The Sergeant washed me down with warm water then examined his handiwork.

'Good, they will have no complaints with that shave.' He sounded proud. As I looked down, I certainly wasn't, it looked revolting. Give me that Black Forest anytime. The nurse now came into her own. She asked me to lift up while she placed a large white sheet under me. Then she painted everywhere that was lily-white with yellow liquid.

'Cor-r! That is cold!' I now looked a state, hairless and bright yellow. She then fastened the sheet on me like a nappy, taped it and said, 'There, all done, they can have you now.'

'Thanks.'

The Sergeant had, in the meantime, departed with his shaving tray only now to return with a needle for me. 'A sharp prick in the arm, then you will feel relaxed and drowsy.' The needle didn't hurt, but nothing seemed to happen. Then, after a little while, my mouth went dry and my eyes a bit heavy. What I didn't feel though, was relaxed. How can anyone feel at ease when you know they are going to cut you up? After a while I was lifted onto a trolley and wheeled away. Only another short journey. This I knew, must be the theatre, or near it. The doctor looked down at me. 'All right Corporal?' I wasn't but nodded bravely.

'I want you to roll over on your side and pull your knees up to your chin. Then I am going to give you an injection in the spine. It will be painful but try to remain still.'

'My God!' It was murder! 'Oh Jesus that hurt,' I was in agony.

'Yes I know. I am sorry, it can't be helped.'

After a while they straightened my legs and eased me onto my back again. The doctor then left the room. I wished I could have gone with him, for I didn't relish my immediate future at all. Drowsiness did begin to creep over me, but not entirely, so that all the time I did have a vague picture of what was happening. The trolley moved again, and then once more I felt myself being lifted. Something was placed over my mouth and lower part of my face. A distant voice told me to breathe deeply. For a second or two I struggled, then relaxed. But I didn't sleep, for as I stared upwards I could see my own body reflected in a myriad of bright lights, not clearly, but as if in a cloud or haze. I closed my eyes and I am convinced I felt for a second, a sensation as if someone had run their fingernail lightly over my groin. After that I remembered nothing.

5

It was as though I had slipped back in time, three years in time, for there I was, listening to those futile words again. 'Take deep breaths, big gulps of air. Come on and you will feel much better.' Bloody rubbish! I was violently sick, I had a terrible headache, and I felt as if someone had impaled me through my back to my front, on a stake. What utter bloody damn fool rubbish! As I came round a little more I found myself lying on my side, staring once more into a vomiting bowl. From the look of it I hadn't just been staring at it either. Beneath the bowl I could see a pair of legs. I glanced upwards to see the nurse. 'Hi, how do you feel now?' As I looked at her I could see I had been sick all over her.

'Sorry,' I said as I flopped back onto the pillow.

'Don't you worry about it.' She wiped my head and face with a cloth. 'I will just go and change, I won't be a minute.' Before she returned, I received two more visitors, the doctor and the Sergeant. I gave them a sickly smile.

The doctor felt my pulse. 'You will be fine now,' then off he went. He could have fooled me. Feel fine! I felt positively like death, and I am sure I must have looked like it. Whilst I had been feeling sorry for myself, the Sergeant had pulled down my sheets and slipped a needle into my backside. I winced but that was all, they could have done what they liked with me, I was too sick to care. Whatever it was it did the trick, and I didn't care for long. Before I knew it I was sound asleep. I must have been that way for hours, for when I eventually opened my eyes it was dusk.

By the light of the lamp above my head, I was able to

take in my surroundings. As I had briefly noticed on my arrival, it was only a small room, with only six beds including mine. The other five were also occupied, four were reading, and one was carefully brushing his hair. Sickness came over me again; I rolled over and started to heave. 'Nurse,' five voices shouted as one. Footsteps, then a cheery, 'Hiya mate.' This from a male nurse with a smile a mile wide. He held the bowl until I had finished.

'Thanks, I feel okay now,' I thought for a while anyway.

'Can I get you something to eat? A piece of toast, a biscuit, anything?'

'No, thanks all the same, although I could murder a cup of tea.'

'Right, give me two minutes.' He looked at the other lads in the ward. 'Come over here you lot and say hello to . . .' he had to hesitate while he looked at my chart, 'to Ray.' The four who had been reading soon slipped off their beds and strolled across. They exchanged brief pleasantries and wished me well, then went back to their books. The hair brushing fifth one didn't come across, but threw a flourishing wave. Please yourself, I thought. My tea arrived, it was perfect. 'Now I want you to drink plenty of water. It is important that you do.' I cut him off short.

'Yes, I know.' The explanation of my plight previously, convinced him that I would co-operate in the object of getting my bladder to fulfil its function.

'Have the lads had a chat?' he asked, smiling.

'All but one, the mermaid there,' for he was still brushing his hair.

'He will be over, don't you fret, his name is Gerald.'

For the first time I noticed the clock on the wall, and I was flabbergasted to find that it said 9.15 p.m. Was it only twelve hours since I called in to the MO that morning? What an eventful day it had been. I wondered if they had informed my Unit where I was, but I wasn't particularly bothered. Apart from my pay that is. I lifted the sheets after a while to see if I could see the extent of my operation. All I could see was the dressing. That reached from beneath

29

my testicles to the top of my hip. I shuddered, but then thought 'well at least it is all over now.' The sheets were still aloft when I felt another pair of eyes staring down.

'Seen enough?' I snapped. For it was our friend Gerald. No wonder I sensed he was there, for he smelt just like a chemist's shop. I stared at him, and had to admit he was most definitely a fine looking bloke. His hair was jet black and beautifully waved. He had light blue eyes and perfect features, but the skin was far too soft-looking for a man. He dropped his hand on mine. It was more like the hand of a woman, long fingered, and I am sure the nails were polished.

'Get off! What game on?' I tried to sit up. 'O-Oh!'

'There, there, I only wanted to comfort you. You don't have to be horrid to me.' The lips pouted as he spoke. It was absolutely incredible, but he was more woman than man.

'I think I like you,' he bent forward, his face close to mine. My eyes frantically looked about, and then looked at my water jug. My fingers had just closed on the handle when, Slap! Gerald suddenly stood erect and tears came flooding to his eyes. Stood behind him was the male night nurse, armed with a tray which had obviously been the weapon he had struck out with.

'Sorry about that. I hoped to be back before he got to be too adventuresome. He always tries it on the new ones.'

'I was getting ready to crown him with my water jug, another minute and he would have had it.'

'So I noticed. My way was more effective, and I can assure you, much more painful.' He sounded very confident.

'By the way, what the heck is he in here for?' I was more than curious.

'Piles!'

I was beginning to feel far from well again with the sickness slowly creeping back over me. So I adopted my usual pose, with my head once more buried deep in a vomiting bowl. That is the position I was still in when the senior night nurse arrived to issue the drugs and injections. He sat on the edge of my bed, checked my pulse, temperature and blood pressure.

30

'Good, you are doing fine. Now I am going to make sure you get a good night's rest. First, drink this.' He handed over a foul concoction. 'Now, roll over.' So yet another needle pierced my backside.

As it turned out, this hospital stay was to be a very, very uneventful one, with just two exceptions. The first of these took place three nights after my arrival. It happened in the dead of night and, to appreciate it, it has to be remembered that one wall was almost a complete window. The lights had been out for at least a couple of hours, but we just couldn't sleep. The moonlight flooded the room with an eerie glow and somehow the shadows seemed to be darker than they should have been. The silence was frightening. It was a very strange feeling, but you could sense we all felt the same. That we knew that the German hospital we shared was an asylum, was something nobody ever seemed to talk about. If I hadn't talked about it before, for some reason I was thinking a lot about it now.

I think I was the first to hear it. It was the creak of a door. Cre—ak. Then silence, but only for a minute. Clonk! Slither! Clonk! Slither! The sound was that of a seemingly heavy footstep immediately followed by what sounded to be the dragging of something heavy. It was obviously coming along the outside passage, whatever it was, and more disconcertingly, it was coming our way.

'What is it?' my voice had more than a tremble in it, for I was situated nearest the door. I looked across at my companions and, like me they had all slid well down in their beds. 'It is all right for you lot, you can bolt for it if you have to, I can't.' Or could I? It might be worth the risk. Then into the room it came. It clonked and slithered over to the window, with the moonlight flinging a huge shadow across the floor and up the wall, a shadow of huge monstrous proportions. Suddenly the ward lights were on.

'Ah, there you are. Come on, they have been looking for you.' There was our monster. A poor little German inmate who, as well as being a bad cripple, wore a large neck and head plaster cast, with his arms outstretched. Our night

31

nurse looked at us and burst out laughing. 'You bloody lot of cowards, you should see your faces. Well I never, the cream of the British Army on the Rhine!' He took the old man's arm. 'Come on Pop, let me take you home.' As he left he turned out the light and laughed, 'Good night children!' There wasn't a murmur; not one of us said a word. Though if they felt like I did, then it was extremely foolish.

The only other thing of importance was the removal of my stitches on the tenth day. I remembered how easy it had been previously at the MRI (Manchester Royal Infirmary), so when the day arrived to do the deed, I was in quite a cocky mood.

'Come on Sergeant, whip them out then I'll be off.'

'Now then, be patient. Don't rush me.' He placed the screens about the bed. I rolled down the bedclothes and undid my pyjama trousers. I lay back and casually placed my hands behind my head, and waited to be told in a few minutes that it was all over. Rip! The plaster had gone. Painful, but not bad. Intense and excruciating pain made my hands shoot up and grab at the bed headrail. I had to grit my teeth to prevent myself crying out in agony. I counted. One, two, three and four onwards until I reached the sum of just fifteen. Fifteen stitches, and every one causing me intense pain. Why the difference, I wondered. The agony I had just suffered, and my vivid recollection from the past when I hadn't felt a thing. Was it 'horses for courses' I wondered, shouldn't nursing be left to women? At that very instance my cry would definitely have been 'Votes for Women'. The following day I was allowed to return to my Unit, clad in my distinctive blue hospital suit, my 'badge of courage'. And so ended another surgical episode.

6

In less than eighteen months I was back in hospital again, this time with a hernia on the other side. I had barely been out of the Army six months and playing cricket this time caused the problem.

The lump had appeared a few weeks before, so consequently my doctor had seen me, and once more I was a surgical case again. Even then, I thought this was a bit much, three spells in three different hospitals, all in less than five years. Anyway I presented myself and felt quite calm and unconcerned. The administration people booked me in, and then I had to wait until another half-dozen men arrived to do the same. We were then gathered together by a blue-uniformed porter, who proceeded to lead us away on what was to be a fairly long route march. He strode majestically ahead, while we all trudged along in his wake. We made our way along a road inside the hospital grounds. Here I kept a wary eye open for passing ambulances! We passed numerous buildings, then entered the main part of the place. It seemed gigantic, the long broad corridor stretching away into the distance. Leading off from this were the wards, some from each side, and they were all three stories high. It certainly meant there were a hell of a lot of patients, no wonder we needed a guide. We eventually reached our destination, block number four. Up one flight of stairs and we were there. The porter handed over his charges to an absolute cracker of a nurse. Dark hair, brown eyes, and even her starchy uniform could not in any way hide her lovely figure. I raised my eyebrows to my companions. This could be very interesting, especially if there were any more like her.

'Good morning gentlemen. Please follow me.' She swayed her way into the ward. Now whether I was the fittest, the youngest or the randiest I don't know, but I was the first behind her!

'Mr Hill, there, the second bed on the right. Get changed and into bed quickly.'

'Yes nurse.' I gave her a mock bow, which she ignored. Moving to the bed she had indicated, I looked at the patients either side of it. Both appeared to be in their sixties. 'Good morning son,' one said, with hand out-stretched. I liked him instantly.

'Morning. Ray's the name.' The man on the other side just rolled and faced the wall, and he sounded as if he was moaning to himself. I quickly stripped off, donned my pyjamas, put away all my things and was about to climb into bed.

'You needn't get into bed yet Mr Hill.' It was the Sister.

'Sorry, the nurse told me to.'

'She would, that's where she likes all her men.' This was said as the nurse returned. As they went away laughing together, it obviously hadn't been a catty remark. Seeing that I did not have to get into the bed, I went for a stroll around the ward. It was a big one indeed, with over thirty beds. It certainly looked a long way from my bed to the toilets and bathroom. I'd have to watch that in case I got taken short. The one thing that I was sorry for was the fact that most of the men really looked ill. So I made my way back, and chatted to my new friend, the old man.

I looked up after being tapped on the shoulder. It was a young doctor. 'Hop into bed please Mr Hill, while I examine you.' I slipped into bed and he drew the curtains. He gave me a thorough check, chest, back, reflexes, blood pressure everything. 'Fine, you are in excellent shape,' he said.

'Oh, can I go then please?'

'Yes, but only when we have pushed your lump back.'

'Ah well, worth a try.'

34

'You will be operated on in the morning sometime, so nothing to eat or drink after tonight's supper.' With that he left me. Sister entered the ward again, this time with a small white-coated orderly.

'Him first, then I will show you the others.'

'Now what,' I wondered.

On his return I knew. Hot water, towels and razor. He looked at my chart. 'Hello Ray. Don't worry, I haven't lost a patient yet, or any part of one for that matter.' I drew the curtains myself before I jumped onto the bed. I slipped off my pyjamas and lay there carefree. He was brilliantly efficient, for even though it wasn't all that long since my last shearing, he really had a lot still to go at. More than it was previously, in fact. I was soon expertly finished, with nary a nick or sign of blood. As he stood back and looked approvingly down, I looked too. And I was very sure that his approving stare was of his handiwork, and not that of nature to me.

The nurse returned, and gave a display of mock shyness. She covered her eyes with her hands. 'Oh, Oh. Will you go and have a bath now. Don't lock the door.' That sounded encouraging! Again, my hopes were dashed. 'If you faint we want to be able to come in and prevent you from drowning,' she hesitated, 'we usually do anyway. Though in your case it might be as well if we left you.' As I walked off with my towel, I chided, 'I love you too.'

Soon back, after a red-hot bath, I was on top of the world. Even my hernia didn't feel so bad. I felt a bit of a fraud really. Time flew by, with interruptions only for meals. I devoured these, as I was ravenous. All good things come to an end though. My end came with the arrival of two nurses who presented themselves just before supper. Their trolley contained a large jug and bowl, and also a length of rubber tubing with a funnel at one end. A frown creased my brow. I was puzzled.

'You're going to love this,' they said.

'Am I?' I had a terrible feeling I wasn't.

'Have you had an enema before?'

35

'A what?'

'Enema, a bowel wash-out. We pour all the water into your tummy, you hold on as long a possible, then dash to the toilet. If you think you can't make it, don't.' She lifted a bedpan. 'You can use this.' It sounded revolting. I looked at the jug. 'I'll never be able to swallow that.'

'You don't have to, it goes in the other end.'

'Oh no, you're not serious!' They both nodded simultaneously.

'Off with your britches and roll over.' I complied, but not happily.

'My God, look at this.' This was the nurse armed with a tube.

'What! Where!' I asked, as my head jerked up.

'Not you,' she said, pushing my head down again. 'You hairy devil, I can't see where to put the bloody thing.' I felt the cheeks of my backside forced open. My head then nearly hit the iron bars at the top of the bed.

'I'll be as gentle as I can,' I was assured. I believed her, but it was a very unpleasant sensation.

'That's it. Now I want you to brace yourself and try and hang on to the water as long as possible. We are going to pour it in now.' My face pressed into the pillow, my fists clenched tightly on the bedsides. I really tried. It wasn't painful by any means, but very unpleasant. I lay there, perspiring and panting as they gaily emptied the contents of the jug down the tube.

'Jesus wept girls. Hurry up please. I know that I am never going to be able to hold on.' I was frantic.

'You can if you try really hard. You pack up too easily.'

'Don't be bloody daft. I am warning you if you don't have that pan ready, there is going to be one hell of a mess. Quickly!' I was very much ashamed of myself, but I was in a state of real panic. Plop! The sensation when the tube came away was a very queasy one. The second it was out, I heaved myself over, and straight onto the bedpan they slipped under me. Splosh! Immediately my cheeks touched it, my bowels were in rapid action. Water flooded out, plus,

I was sure, my liver, intestines and kidneys as well. Also, I was in trouble.

'You should hold on to it longer than that, otherwise the exercise is futile,' I was admonished with a wagging finger.

'Futile my foot! If I had false teeth, they would have been in the pan as well as everything else.'

'Alright then, off you get while we clean you up.' I rolled over, and off the foul-smelling heap, and flopped face down. Exhausted.

They both set to and washed my backside with gusto, towelled me, and finally powdered me with a flourish. Now this bit I liked.

'There, now you are presentable again.' I felt it, and smelt it!

'Drinks will be along soon. Remember, one only, then absolutely nothing else at all.' With that, they took away my water jug and glass. A stern reminder of tomorrow.

'Right sir!' I saluted. The wet sponge caught me full in the face. As if on cue, the Sister walked through the curtains.

The thrower, unabashed, turned to her and said, 'I think we are going to have trouble here.'

'I have a terrible feeling you are right. But not for two or three days at least,' then after a second, 'or perhaps longer if I have a word with the anaesthetist.' Then they all left before the drinks came along. I had a cup of tea, snuggled down, and immediately went to sleep.

'Wake up. Come on wake up.' I had been in a deep sleep. 'I want you to swallow this tablet, so you will have a good night's sleep.' I heard the voice, but as yet couldn't see its owner. I rolled over and sat bolt upright.

'How daft can you bloody be? Fancy waking me up to give me a sleeping pill!' Facing me was a lady, the night Sister, and she must have been nearing the end of her career. Her hair was iron grey, and her eyes looked tired. Instinct told me to apologise, and quickly! I was too late.

'Who do you think you are talking to. I am old enough to be your mother, and don't swear at me again or I will . . .'

she changed her mind. A quick belt on the head with my chart from the bottom of my bed. 'Or I will do that.'

'Ouch! I am very sorry but I was sound asleep. You must admit it does sound a bit barmy.' I never learn. Bang!

'Swallow this and shut up. I will decide what is barmy and what is not.'

What ensued the following day with little variation (except I had no one to salute) was a repeat of my last 'hernia' operation. Knees bent, then wham! It was like being hit with a cannonball, but this time sleep came as well.

My return from the land of nod was also identical, with the violent sickness playing the all-important part. We had two days of that, but once it stopped I started to improve at once. Even the stitch removal went smoothly, eighteen and not one felt, for it was the tender hand and expertise of Sister. Lord be praised for lady nurses. Obviously, before I left I blotted my copybook. There had been too many really sick elderly people to allow any frivolity at all. I appreciated this and conducted myself accordingly, except just for one time.

The poor old chap next to me on my left, the one who had been gently moaning to himself when I arrived, had slowly but surely deteriorated as the days went by. In spite of all the hard work, attention, devotion and brilliant nursing, the poor old fellow just passed away. It happened in the early hours of the morning, so with all the activity going on around him I was lying awake. It was then that I saw the seamier side of hospital life and death. It was when I heard the crying and anguish of his family, that the thought crossed my mind. Is it worth the fighting, the futile fighting, when all the effort only seemed to prolong what was surely the inevitable. Why couldn't they be allowed to help him to die sooner, and much more peacefully, for both his, and his relatives' sakes?

The following morning the adjoining bed was empty and newly made up, ready for new arrivals. Soon after nine o'clock the nurse arrived with a new batch of patients. She pointed to the bed, and directed one of the victims in its direction. Which as it turned out, was my direction also.

'Morning,' I said in a cheerful voice and offered my hand.

'Hello.' It was an obviously nervous reply. Just at that moment Sister passed by for the first time that morning.

'Good morning Mr Smith. Mr Hill will help you settle in, won't you?' How could I resist such a threat?

'What are you in for, a little or a lot?' I rolled over to face him.

'I have a hernia,' he replied, not happily.

'Don't worry about that, I have had two of them,' I told him cockily. 'At least with that there is no chance of you popping off like the last occupant of that bed.' I knew at once that I had put my foot in it, for he immediately stood up and looked down at the bed.

'Here?'

I nodded gravely.

'When?'

'Early this morning. It was very sad.' I really meant it.

He looked very pale and far from happy. Then he asked, 'Is there another Mr Smith in here?' and looked about the ward.

'Not now there isn't, that was him who had that bed.' To my amazement he immediately scuttled out of the ward. Funny fellow, I thought to myself. He returned shortly, accompanied by the Sister. She stared at me haughtily.

'I will see you later,' she snapped. They gathered his things together, and moved to the top of the ward. The landing of a pillowcase full of newly laundered crepe bandages on the end of my bed heralded her return.

'Roll those.' She was livid.

'What have I done?' I asked.

'For your information, the late Mr Smith was his uncle.'

'Enough said.' I settled down to my bandage rolling. Two days later I was discharged.

7

Just less than five years rolled by before I was forced to return to the hospital scene. As well as a change of venue, it was also a change of complaint. A battered nose! This was the result of two collisions between the same nose and a couple of cricket balls. As the latter were without doubt the harder, the nose definitely came off second best. Bent and broken! Breathing was a problem, with the added complication of sinus trouble. Before they decided to operate, they tried a few excursions up my nasal passages with pointed sticks and syringes. This was not at all to my liking. It was messy and it was painful, and while you were having the treatment you sat in waiting rooms like well-tusked elephants. As the treatment was not very successful, it was decided that I would have to spend a few days in hospital, the Ear, Nose and Throat Hospital. Five days at most, I was told. This meant it couldn't be much of a thing, so I was happy enough to present myself to get the thing over with.

The hospital and its wards were very small, but the oddest thing to me was how strangely quiet it was. Though on more reflection that was understandable, for with a bad throat you couldn't speak, with bad ears you couldn't hear, and with a bad nose you couldn't breathe properly. If you can't breathe properly, you can't talk much. So hence the quietness!

I was examined quickly by a German lady doctor, who pricked and prodded up my nose with a torch type of probe. I didn't like it very much.

'Well I think we can clear this up for you, Mr Hill. You see, what we will do is to chip all the damaged bone away

40

to clear the passages. What we can't do for you is to straighten your nose.' Chip it away! She made me sound like a piece of granite, and she a sculptor. Though that could about sum it up, for she was built like a brickie. I hope she doesn't blame me for losing the war.

'I am not particular about the appearance of the nose, and it is immaterial to me in which direction it points, just so long as it functions properly.' I was deadly serious, because not long before, I had nearly gassed myself, and it was that instance that had made me seek help in the first place.

The following day it was business as usual. Early rising, no food or drink and, as I didn't sport a moustache there was, for a change, no shaving to be done. It wasn't long before I was shunted into the theatre for the deed to be done. I was fitted with a skullcap and a sheet wrapped around my neck. A set-up, I thought, more in keeping with a woman having a facial than me having a bit of an operation. They gave me a local anaesthetic in the nose and left me for a while. Soon I was on the move again, though this time not far. Just a few inches up the table it was, and then my head back to leave my nostrils pointing skywards. I wouldn't say I found the prospect of someone going to belt away at me with a hammer and chisel hilarious, so I kept my eyes tightly shut, and wished I could do the same with my ears. Tap. Tap. Tap. To my utter amazement I didn't feel a thing, and I only heard the faintest of noise. Then in no time at all, it was all over. I was soon back in the ward and tucked into bed. There was a small dressing taped under my nose, and that was all. The thing that pleased me the most was the fact that there was no sickness, just a foul taste in the mouth, and that I was quite happy to put up with. I felt I could tolerate anything rather than have to face up to the heaving I had done in the past.

There was no trouble this time with the bowels, bladder or stitches. It was, apart from a pretty constant drip of blood from the beak, a fairly uneventful excursion into the realms

41

of hospital life. Things gradually dried up, and I was able to breathe better than I had for many a month. Obviously the thing had been a big success, so on the fifth day I was discharged.

8

Two years later I had to make a brief visit to another hospital, on the outskirts of Manchester this time. So yet again it was another change of surroundings.

For some time, my wife and I had had some difficulty in conceiving a child, so it was decided that I should have some kind of a test to check the possibility that this was due to a failing on my part. What they were going to do to me, I had no idea. I imagined all kinds of painful injections or some such terrible things. I reported to the hospital at ten thirty in the morning, and was directed to the Pathological Laboratory. As I approached the tiny window I was shattered to see a really smart blonde girl who must have only been in her early teens.

'Yes sir, can I help you?' she asked sweetly.

I hesitated, then stammered, 'Here is my doctor's letter.' She took it and moved away from the window for a moment or two. On her return she wrote my name on the label of a small brown bottle.

'Here you are Mr Hill, will you go along the passage there to the toilet, and let me have a specimen.' I looked at the bottle. It was so tiny. 'A specimen of my water in there? Do you want it as I start, in the middle or as I'm finishing?' I held up the bottle to her. 'Let's face it, it will only hold a drop of water.'

'I don't want water Mr Hill,' she said calmly. The penny dropped. 'Oh no!' I thought to myself, 'it can't be this way, not in this day and age.' As I looked into her eyes I could see it was. My blush as I made my way to the toilet, reached from the top of my shirt collar to my receding hairline.

I entered the toilet and slammed the door behind me, flopping down on the seat. I sat staring at the bottle in my hand. Bloody hell! What a bloody performance, what a stupid sodding arrangement. I was furious with the hospital, my own doctor and most of all, myself. Fancy letting myself be talked into this, I must be crazy.

At last, I calmed down. Well you're here lad, and you had better do what is expected of you and get on with it. I undid my zip, and withdrew the doubtful object that had led me to this predicament. It hung there limp, and looked ever so pathetic. Masturbation! It was something I had never felt the urge to do in my life, even in my early adolescence. Well come on, get on with it then. I took hold of the thing and tried. For a few minutes I tried, but nothing happened. So I tried with the other hand for a few minutes more. Still nothing! Closing my eyes, I tried to think of everything that could possibly turn me on. I concentrated hard. Now try again lad. A light grip and once more I was off. Come on lad, try harder still. As I stood there now, sweating profusely, I thought, why the hell don't they provide you with a 'sexy' book to read at the same time as they give you the diminutive little bottle to fill. How the hell they expected a man to sexually stir himself, locked alone in a bare hospital toilet, devoid of even such a thing as a VD poster, I'll never know. The thought crossed my mind to go back to the girl in the window and beg her assistance, but I thought better of it. Suddenly, something stirred. Now it had started it came with a bloody rush. Christ! What do I do now? I grabbed for the bottle at the back of the toilet seat. How stupid could I be, I had not taken the top off the damn thing. Somehow I managed it with one hand and my teeth. By this time I was nearly on my knees with exhaustion. I sagged wearily onto the seat, still keeping a firm grip on my manhood. I somehow managed to collect some of the requested, and hard won sample of my hopefully reproductive fluid.

I sat there for a while, then cleaned myself up as best I

could, then I noticed there, on the back of the door, a notice that made me smile to myself. It read:

In the interest of hygiene
Please wash your hands.

Going through to the washroom I did as the notice instructed, and gave myself a thorough clean up.

Now what! How the heck can I go back and face that young girl? How can I walk up to her with my small bottle as if I hadn't a care in the world? Do I go out looking as embarrassed as I really felt, or do I put on a front and cheek it out? I chose the latter.

Striding down the corridor, I slammed the bottle down. 'Here you are love,' staring her straight in the face.

'Thank you Mr Hill.'

'It was my pleasure!' I replied. I turned on my heels and strode out of the place. Quickly.

9

The years went by very actively. I worked and played hard, being very much involved in football, cricket and table tennis. Slowly, I began to notice that I had a constant companion, both during, and after my sporting excursions. This was a painful left knee. It started just by being rather troublesome, but gradually it deteriorated, becoming a very frustrating and bloody nuisance, niggling away at the joint like a severe toothache.

At first, I thought steadfastly, no hospital this time that's for sure, so I took myself to an osteopath who had a fine reputation in the area. A true and honest man, he told me after a few visits that it was something that he could not cure. He advised me to see an orthopaedic surgeon. It was some months before I took his advice, saw my own doctor, and eventually found myself in yet another hospital, my fifth. I arrived at the ward around Sunday lunchtime, and for the first time, entered the orthopaedic world. Immediately it felt so much different, it had an atmosphere all of its own.

A nurse quickly took me into the ward where I undressed and packed my things away in my grip for my wife to take away with her. We didn't know it then, but this situation was going to develop into a regular habit. I lay on top of the bed and gazed around the ward. The first thing that impressed me was the lack of neat military precision as far as the beds were concerned. Beds, in my previous hospital stays, had always been neatly made with immaculate and straight counterpanes. Pillows also, had always been tucked away tidily behind the patients. Here it seemed as if all the occupants of the ward had been involved in a gigantic pillow fight. Sheets and counterpanes had the appearance of being thrown over the beds any old how. The more you looked, and the more you noticed the varying shapes that occupied the beds, the more you realised it was virtually impossible to keep a bed tidy for long.

There were limbs slung high, wide and handsome, some in plaster, and some not. Legs were also stretched over the end of the beds with weights dangling from them. This, to me had a slight medieval torture look. Arms also were extended in plaster casts in various and strange positions, looking like branches on windblown trees. The rest of the beds seemed to all be mushroom-shaped at the ends. This, I discovered, was the shape of metal cages that kept the weight of the bedclothes off damaged limbs.

As I became more accustomed to my surroundings, another important thing impressed me, and that was the noise, the noise of laughter. To my ears, the majority of the patients appeared to be laughing or chatting away quite merrily. This sound really and truly appealed to me, and I joined in at the first opportunity.

The day passed quickly by, and I made the late night drinks at the request of the nurse. My tea and coffee I could recommend, but my milk drinks, such as Horlicks, Ovaltine etc., I couldn't, for the life of me, master. There were more lumps in it than army gravy. Like the kind soul I was, I collected and washed up the cups and saucers, at the same time making the nurse and myself a few rounds of toast and jam. The Lord helps those who help themselves.

At the unearthly hour of 5.30 a.m., I was awakened by the steady drip of cold water on my face. I half opened my eyes to see, poised above me, my water jug with water gently dripping out onto my face. It was held, very sadistically, by the night nurse. In moving to take evasive action, I jumped too quickly and too high, and caught the jug on the top of my head. It went up and over backwards. The result was one very surprised and wet young lady.

'Bloody hell, I didn't expect that.'

'Sorry love, here let me wipe you dry.' I picked up my towel.

'No thanks.' She stepped back quickly as I moved forward. For it was her chest that had taken the full force of the water, and for some strange reason, she didn't seem to want me to rub her bosom. Why, at five thirty in the morning, I'll never know! I went along to the kitchen, made the tea for the lads, and then trundled my way into the ward.

'Wakey! Wakey!' a bit noisy it sounded, but I was competing with clanging bowls and jugs, plus a few good lusty 'Woodbine' coughs.

'Tea lads. Speak now, or forever hold your peace. No not that one!' I quickly circulated with my trolley, and satisfied the wants (within reason of course) of my fellow sufferers. The pots washed once again, I started to leave the kitchen, but I was collared before I had gone two steps.

'Will you help with the breakfast trays please.' This, from the orderly who had arrived from another ward, and was busily buttering bread.

'No,' I said as I swiped a lovely brown crust. Out I went once again on my rounds. The good thing about this was that it enabled me to settle at once into the fellowship of the ward, and immediately become a part of the 'family'. For already, in just over half a day, I had spoken to more people than in the full five days of my last hospital stay. Having completed my mission, I returned to the kitchen with my empty vehicle.

'You're a dish, Mr Hill,' the nurse told me.

'I know!'

After a quick wash and shave, I lay on my bed, reading and listening to the music on my earphones. I had an excellent breakfast, followed by a little kip.

'Wake up Mr Hill, ward round.' I was being gently shaken. The surgeon and his cronies were already half-way round the room by the time I had pulled myself together. When it was my turn, Sister introduced me.

'This is Mr Hill, sir.'

'Ah yes, the mystery knee.' He turned to his followers. As he talked about me, I heard him using the words 'it could be' and 'it might also be this,' and I began to have doubts. Seemingly, he didn't.

'Don't worry, we will sort it out for you.' I wished I could be sure. When they had gone, Sister returned, and on seeing the obvious look of doubt on my face, sat on the end of my bed.

'The knee is a strange joint, and takes a tremendous amount of wear and tear. Also, in lots of cases, we cannot tell, until we see inside the actual joint, the really true picture. But rest assured, they will put you right.'

'When will that be?' I asked.

'Tomorrow morning, early,' she told me, 'the girls will prep you later today.'

A few games of cards and dominoes made the day move along at a fast pace, so that it was late afternoon when two young nurses summoned me from a game.

'Mr Hill, come along while we prepare you for the big day.'

'Right girls, just a minute and I will be with you.' I then strolled away to the sluice.

'Charming!'

My curtains were drawn when I got back. I entered my harem; the nurses were sat on my bed.

'Do you feel better now?' they asked together. I nodded as I sprawled on the bed.

'Put this on, then we will shave you,' the senior girl said, as she threw at me a white piece of material with a small tape at each corner.

'What is it, and where do I put it?' I asked, holding it aloft.

'It is a 'fig-leaf' and you put it where your pyjama pants are now.' She took it off me, opened her legs wide, and said 'like this.' I untied my pyjamas.

'No peeking!' I said, as I slipped them off. I then tied on my nappy, for that is what it reminded me of. They certainly weren't tailored by Hardy Amis, that was for sure. Fortu-

49

nately, they weren't a bad fit, for too small would most certainly have cut you in half, whereas too large would see the whole thing slipping down over the hips every time you moved an inch. Standing back to look at me, they talked about me, and not to me.

'I think he looks like Hiawatha,' said one.

'No,' said the other as she stood back to look, 'no, I know who he reminds me of.' She turned and took off the trolley a tin of Johnson's baby powder, 'Him!'

'Have you done, you two? It is not very nice of you to insult and upset me when I am poorly in hospital.' I lay back and took up a pose of agony and despair. At that precise moment, Sister entered.

'How are things progressing in here? My God, are you alright, Mr Hill?' moving forward quickly. I sat up quicker!

'Sorry Sister, just a bit of play acting for the sake of your protégés here.' It must have been a good performance to fool her, if only for a second or two. The same protégés were now busily placing a large towel under me, prior to the shaving.

'I see, I see. But come on, we must get on, for there is a lot more work to do.' Then she herself commenced the application of the soapy lather, all over the front of my leg. Her next words took me completely by surprise, as I am convinced she meant them to.

'You shave him nurse, there always has to be a first time, and it might as well be now.' As the nurse picked up the razor, and moved forward, somewhat shakily, I mentally gave the first round to Sister. She watched carefully that the poor young girl didn't do the surgeon's job for him. When she was satisfied that I would keep my leg, she left them to it. The final hairless, smooth skin that was left after the young nurse's first attempt at shaving, was a credit to her. There they were, side by side, one absolutely bare and devoid of even one hair, and the other looking like a rolled up coconut mat. As they packed up their things, they told me to go along and have a bath.

On my return from the bathroom I was told to get into

bed and stay there. A sudden thought crossed my mind, and not a happy one at that. When would I have my enema? The thought of it even made me sweat a bit. I lay there in bed reading to pass the time now I was supposedly to be incarcerated in it. But every time I heard the wheels of a trolley I shuddered, expecting to see the jug, tube and funnel that would herald a bowel 'de-coke'.

The day staff left after we had had our supper, to be replaced by the same night staff as the previous evening.

'What am I going to do without you, Mr Hill?' wailed the nurse.

'Ah well, I am poorly now. I wasn't last night, but I am now.' I went into my dying swan routine.

'Oh my God!' the nurse laughed, 'stay like that and I will be back in just one minute.' True to her word she was. She started to draw my curtains.

'What now?' I asked.

'You'll see, I won't be a minute.' Then I heard the clatter of the trolley wheels. Here it comes, I told myself. It did, but no instruments of torture did I see on it.

'Where are they then?' I could see the bedpan, a pair of thin rubber gloves, and what looked like two silver bullets, and that was all.

'Where are what?'

I explained about my previous enema.

'We don't do that here. Roll over and leave your bum facing me.' I complied with the request. 'Now I am going to push two suppositories as far as I can, then I want you to hold on as long as you are able. Then shout when you want the pan.'

'Can't I sit on it as soon as they are in?' I asked.

'No, you will cheat that way. You have to sit tight for as long as you can manage. Ready? Oh just a minute, I can't see a damn thing here.' The sound of scissors clipping away came from my stern area.

'What the hell are you doing?' I turned sharply to see what she was up to. 'Bloody Nora!' the point of the scissors stuck into my arse!

51

'Serves you right. Keep still, it is bad enough cutting this imitation privet hedge without you rolling all over the place. Now lie still. Are you ready, here they come.' I think she was enjoying herself. I felt the thing slip inside, then felt her finger push the object as far as she could. She then repeated the performance.

'Good, now try and hold them for as long as you can.'

'You won't go far will you?' I looked round for the bedpan. 'Put that thing where I can get at it. What if you are on the loo or something? I will be a dead duck.'

'I can always change the bed,' and off she went.

I lay there, face downwards, not daring to move. Oh my God, where is she? 'Nurse!' at the top of my voice.

'Hold on Mr Hill, I am busy,' her voice came from the other end of the ward. Oh no! She must come; I could feel the thing building up inside me.

'Oh nurse, where are you?' I was getting desperate, 'Nurse!' Then I leapt out of bed and made a bolt for the sluice. I passed her on her way to me, but I didn't stop! Just in time, I slammed my behind down on a seat. What a clear out! It was long, it was loud, and very smelly!

Knock, knock!

'Mr Hill? Raymond, why didn't you wait until I could bring you a bedpan? You are not supposed to be out of bed,' she was furious, 'do you want to get me into trouble?'

'Now, now nurse, don't change the subject,' I chided her.

'Come on you fool, get back into bed. Then I will come along and wash your feet.'

'Oh Jesus!' This as I opened the toilet door, and strode past her in my bare feet.

'Don't be blasphemous, or I will stamp on your toes.' It was only when I heard the catcalls from the other occupants of the ward as we entered, that I realised what a case I must have looked. For remember, I had on a pyjama top, my fig leaf, and that was all. As I padded along, I laughed as I realised what a sight I must have presented as I made my belt for the sluice!

Back in bed, I waited for my feet to be washed. The

nurse brought a bowl and quickly cleaned them up. As she finished I rested my hand gently on her head.

'Thank you my child,' I said in a deep solemn voice. And then I crossed myself.

'That is enough. There are some very religious men in here.' She left me to go and make the supper drinks, which she had soon distributed. I enjoyed two sweet cups of tea, and then settled down for a read. As the nurse collected the cups, she said, 'Remember, no more to drink, now, or in the morning.' She also removed my water jug. The night Sister arrived, gave me a knockout drop, and I was soon away.

I didn't seem to have been asleep for more than a few minutes before I was being shaken awake! I had a good wash and shave, then immediately settled down and fell asleep again.

The next time I was disturbed it was by the Staff Nurse who had arrived with a trolley.

'Wakey, wakey, Mr Hill, prep time.' She rolled down the sheets and painted my leg a beautiful shade of pink, then wrapped it up and taped it securely for the theatre. She then gave me a clean fig leaf and 'back to front' nightie.

'There you are, all ready for the off. All you need is your pre-med. injection in a few minutes, then they can have you.' As good as her word, she was back in a few minutes with the needle. She was competent, for I didn't feel a thing.

It was not long after my mouth had dried up completely, that my charioteer arrived to drive me to the theatre. He would have done credit to a 'whiter than white' commercial. White skullcap, mask, shirt and trousers. I could compete with him quite well, especially my face! For as I slid off my bed onto his trolley, I was more than a bit scared. He stopped outside the Sister's office.

'Don't worry Mr Hill, I am sending a pretty nurse with you to hold your hand!' She did too, for the girl that went along with me was quite a corker.

The journey wasn't long, and I was wheeled into the anaesthetist's room, adjacent to the theatre. As I looked up at the gentleman who was to prepare me for the Surgeon, I just didn't know what to expect. All too well, I remembered the spinal injections of the past, and hoped it would not be a similar thing. I was lucky.

'Hello, Mr Hill. This is quite simple and, I assure you, quite painless.' He seemed sincere anyway. 'Just a needle in the back of your hand, and you will be away.'

'Right.' I sounded like I felt. Relieved!

'Here we go,' he said. I watched the needle as it went in. He was right, I hardly felt it. I continued to watch it until he told me to start counting from one to ten. Backwards.

'Ten, nine, eight, sev . . .,' the needle disappeared, and so did all my faculties. I was away. Well away.

As usual, on my return to the land of the living I was in my customary position. Head in a receiving bowl, and being as sick as a dog.

'O-o-oh.' I felt terrible, or at first I thought I did. Then, as just a little time went by, and the initial sickness left me, I came to realise that I didn't feel too bad at all. I felt strange, indeed I couldn't understand it. Only the faintest sign of sickness, no perspiring, and no pain at all in the leg. Now that was the puzzling part, why no pain? As I lay there, I couldn't understand this at all. Slowly, I slid my hand down my leg to feel for plaster, bandages or whatever. But I could feel nothing, absolutely nothing.

'Nurse!' I shouted. 'Nurse!' I howled, louder this time.

'Are you fully awake now Mr Hill? We have been waiting for you to come completely to your senses, because Sister wants to talk to you.' The poor nurse was itching to get away. 'I will go and tell her you are awake.'

'Tell her that I am very much awake, and I want to see her more than she wants to see me.' I was shouting as she left.

Sister marched in, followed by the nurse.

'Now Mr Hill, calm down and I will explain to you what has happened. Or more to the point, what hasn't happened. But before I do I want you to apologise to this nurse for shouting at her.'

'Alright, I am really sorry, but you must admit, it is a bit

54

of a shock.' I looked at them inquisitively. 'What went wrong?' Sister sat down on the edge of my bed.

'Well they think they know what is wrong with your knee, but there is just a little doubt about it, so they are going to do it next week instead.' I sat there flabbergasted.

'I don't believe you.'

'It is true Mr Hill. The knee is a very tricky joint and they must be absolutely sure exactly where they go in.' Bewildered, I could only stare at her in disbelief. I shook my head a few times, and then finally accepted the situation.

'What do I do now then?' I asked.

'You can go home in the morning, then I want you back here on Sunday afternoon.' She stood up to leave. 'How would you like some tea and toast?'

'Yes please.' Well why not, I thought.

I went home on the Wednesday, and subsequently went back to work, a surprise both to the neighbours and my colleagues in the mill.

The time soon came to return to the hospital, it still seemed farcical to me but there it was. I reported to the ward and popped my head in the office.

'Good afternoon Sister,' I said cheerfully, thinking I had better start off on the right foot.

'Ah, Mr Hill, good afternoon.' She beckoned me forward. 'Come on in.' Now what? I might be suspicious, but something else was wrong, I knew it.

'We have a minor problem, there is no bed for you in the ward. Wait before you go off half-cocked,' she lifted her hand to stop my outburst, 'but we have you a bed in our single private ward at the end of the corridor.'

'I don't really fancy that much.' I would rather have been with men in the general ward.

'It is that or nothing I'm afraid.'

'OK I give in, lead me to it.' I picked up my bag and opened the door. The Sister showed me the room. If you really liked to be alone it was ideal, not too small, and with its own wash-basin and mirror. But not for me, for I like to chatter!

'I can tell you are not thrilled at the idea, so I promise you the minute there is a bed vacant, I will move you to the ward.' I couldn't complain at that, so I made myself at home.

The following day, and up to my pre-med. time on the Tuesday morning, it was just a repeat of the previous week. The one exception being that a leg shave was not required, only a fresh coat of pink paint. Sister came along to give me my injection.

'Here we go again.' I couldn't resist it.

'Rest assured, all will be well this time,' she promised. 'Also, when you wake up, you will be in the main ward.' I was really pleased at the news.

'Oh thanks Sister.' My driver and nurse came for me again, and we made our journey together for the second time.

I opened my eyes and stared at the ceiling. Immediately I knew. Slight sickness but no pain! My mouth opened wide.

'Sister!' I yelled. My hand felt all around my knee. It was sore, but that was all.

'Sister!' I yelled even louder, and sat up in bed. She had kept her promise, I was in the ward. I looked for sympathy from my companions.

'They have done it again,' I shouted at them. I could tell they all knew!

Sister arrived, accompanied by a doctor. He was still attired in his surgical theatre kit. They drew the curtains about us.

'Now what?' I wasn't happy at all. 'Did you lose the knife?' As soon as I said it, I apologised. 'Sorry.'

'That is understandable, don't apologise. But you must understand our position with your knee, we must be absolutely sure. At first we thought it was a piece of bone chipped off, though now we are not satisfied, so we are going to try something else.' Give them their due, they certainly did try!

I was discharged from the ward, and then had to return in a few days as an 'out-patient'. This was a brand new experience for me in my medical history. It was June 1961,

56

and it was also my first excursion into the world of physio-therapy. It was a world that I was going to become very, very familiar with in the years to come.

I was taken, by a smart young girl, into a small cubicle. I removed my trousers on request, lay on the couch, and watched her as she manoeuvred an infra-red heat lamp into position. She situated it just above the knee, turned it on and left me with the words:

'If it gets too hot give me a shout.' A few minutes later she was back to turn off the power.

'You can go now Mr Hill.'

'Is that it?' I asked.

'Yes that's it. Three times a week we want to see you.' I honestly couldn't, for the life of me, see this being the answer, but they knew best. Or so I hoped!

When two weeks had gone past with my six visits, I had to return to the hospital to see the surgeon. I reported no change in my condition; the knee was just as bad as ever. So it was back to the physio again. The treatment was slightly different on this occasion. Different cubicle, differ-ent lamp, it was ultra-violet this time. The time under it was very quickly over, it seemed only seconds.

Another two weeks went by, and all I had to show for it was a two-inch square of sun-tanned skin. No relief of the pain at all, just a very brown piece of skin. Back once more to the surgeon.

Again I reported no improvement. The joint was exam-ined thoroughly once more; it was getting to be very habit forming. I was then told that I was going to have a hydro-cortisone injection. Sublimely innocent of what to expect, I was taken into another room. I removed my trousers (yet again, a female request), then lay there, calmly waiting for the doctor. Two nurses assisted him; one rubbed the knee with an antiseptic solution, while the other passed him a large needle. Feeling around the joint on the inside of the leg, he found the troublesome spot.

'There it is, am I right?' he asked. The damn fool only had to look at my face to know. Even as I looked, in went the needle! Apart from the fact that the bloody thing must have transfixed me to the table, I felt sure I would have rebounded from the ceiling. Never in my life had I experienced such pain. The nearest to it, being the lumbar punctures in the past. It was excruciating.

'No cricket or table tennis, nothing that affects the knee. Avoid kneeling also, and I will see you in a month.' I was going to ask if I should walk on my hands, but thought better of it, so I left the place bitterly disappointed. Deep down I knew that this wasn't the answer.

Returning after another month had passed, with no change at all, they decided to give me another injection. It seemed even worse this time, for I knew what to expect, and I didn't like it. Two weeks later, I was discharged and told to rest the knee as much as possible. They wrote to my doctor and that was that. What a farce.

10

1964, and the knees are far from good. Yes, it is pain in the plural now. The left knee joint was by far the worst, but I wasn't yet to realise that the other wasn't very far behind in the 'surgery stakes'.

Since my last fruitless hospital visits, I had moved home, and subsequently changed my doctor. It didn't take him long to decide that I could be a good candidate for a National Health Service holiday. He told me, 'Well, there is something wrong with the joints, but I personally don't know what. So I am going to send you to someone who will.' I was sceptical.

'I have heard all that before, as you can see from my notes.'

'This will be different, I assure you.' He sounded very confident. So, as I had a very high regard for his medical opinion, I left his surgery feeling on top of the world!

It took more than a little time to finally get an appointment with the orthopaedic surgeon, but at last my time came, and off to the hospital I went. As I made my way through the gates at the entrance, my thoughts went way back to that time when I had passed through them as a teenager. I carefully poked my head round the corner before I decided to venture across the yard. This time I was lucky, there were no dashing ambulances.

Making my way into the large hall, I was pleased to see a great many changes. Plush red chairs, bright coloured walls, and even a number of fish tanks. The long hours of waiting also seemed a thing of bygone ages, for an efficient system kept the patients moving through the clinic at a very steady rate. This did away with the hours of impatient and agonising boredom.

'Mr Hill, please.' The sound of my name echoed around the hall, as the nurse spoke into a small microphone fastened to the wall. Another innovation. I stood, forcing myself up out of the deep armchair with effort. All eyes seemed to focus on me as I threaded my way past a sea of 'plasters'. There were leg plasters, arm plasters, crutches and walking sticks. If you didn't have a broken leg when you entered the place, it was almost certain you would have one by the time you reached the doctor. Eventually, I made my goal.

'This way Mr Hill,' the nurse said politely. She then led me to a curtained cubicle.

'Off with your shoes, socks and trousers, then lie on the bed.' I complied with her wishes. As I lay there looking around me I little knew how many times that I was to be there in those surroundings.

Approaching footsteps heralded the arrival of the surgeon. He was a fine military looking man who I instantly took a liking to. Efficiency literally oozed out of him. For that reason I felt confident immediately.

'Hello Mr Hill, what seems to be the trouble?' he asked. The voice was firm but pleasant. I began to relate the history of the left, and then the right knee so far. While he listened, he was giving the joints a very thorough workout. He bent, straightened and twisted the legs in all the positions imaginable, and also in some that weren't. I ooed and ahd in as quiet a tone as possible. It was a necessary, if unpleasant experience. The climax of it came when he gently pressed the kneecap down against the joint, and rotated it slowly. My eyeballs also rotated. He had really found the trouble spots.

'That certainly made me squirm a bit,' I told him.

'I thought it might.' He turned to the nurse. 'Send him for an x-ray then I will see him again later.' A nod and a smile, and he was off seeing the rest of the patients.

I was given directions to find the x-ray department, which

I did by simply following the signs and arrows. Here I had my first pictures of knees. I didn't know then how photogenic they were going to be. The lady called me in.

'Take off your trousers,' she told me. For the number of times over the following years that I was told that, I could have practically bought my suits with no trousers at all.

I got on the table, then it was, 'Knee bent, lie still.' Click. 'Now left side, still.' Click. 'Right side, still.' Click. The studio session over, I returned with my plates to the surgeon. I sat and waited for just a little while, and then I was seen again. He examined the x-ray plates on the machine, nodded his head, and turned to me.

'Yes Mr Hill, you will have to come into us and we will scrape the back of your patella.' He seemed so matter of fact.

'Scrape my patella?' I wasn't even sure what it was, though I had guessed that it must be my kneecap. Scrape the back of them, it sounded horrific. How the hell do you get to the back of them? That it scared me obviously showed in my face.

'Don't worry, we are doing it all the time,' he told me. Not wanting to show the fear that both he and I knew I felt, I didn't even ask how, why, or even when. I just slipped on my clothes and left.

Months went by, with the knees becoming more and more painful as the time passed. Then at last the hospital thankfully summoned me to join them, and wasn't I glad they did. I didn't really care what they did to me, just as long as it wasn't going to be another repetition of the 'shall we, shan't we' episode I had previously experienced.

I was booked in at the main office. Name, address and next of kin (an unfair question this of anybody going into hospital. It didn't fill you with confidence at all!). These details completed, I was led, with some others, to the ward. A long route march to S1. This ward was quite large and was situated on both sides of the main corridor. There was a long side and then a much shorter one, plus a couple of side wards. With the ward situated as it was, it seemed to be very, very busy, with a steady movement of people to and fro. Nurses, orderlies, physios and patients, on trolleys and off them.

'It's like bloody Piccadilly Circus isn't it?' I said to my companions. At that precise moment, and before anyone could answer me, the 'bloody' part seemed to be right. A stretcher appeared off the corridor, being carried into the ward, and alongside it marched a nurse carrying a bottle of blood held high, to enable it to drip down the tube to the arm that was lying limp on the stretcher. I was extremely glad when the nurse led us to the opposite side of the corridor and into the ward.

My bed was at the far end of the ward, the last on the left. This in itself was a complete change, for usually in my stays I had always been the first on the right. Was this a good sign? I thought. I was soon undressed and in bed like the well-trained patient that I was. I turned to my neighbour, 'Good morning,' I said cheerfully. The only answer I received was a positive grunt of unfriendliness. 'Get stuffed!' I said to myself.

As I looked around, there was the usual array of plaster casts, legs, arms and spikers, plus a lot of sad, head injury cases. It was, in some of these cases, very upsetting to see the men sitting and just staring ahead but seeing nothing. My complaint seemed again, so trivial that somehow I felt guilty about taking the bed. I consoled myself with the thought that these people couldn't afford the time to attend to me if they didn't really think it was a necessity. I didn't have any more chance to feel sorry for myself, because then a young doctor arrived.

'Morning Mr Hill,' as he pulled the curtains.

'Good morning Doctor,' I said politely.

'First, I want your full medical history, and then I want to give you a thorough examination. OK?'

'Fine by me.' I pointed to my nose, 'Shall we start here,' then pointing to my knees, 'or here?'

'Let us start from the top,' he said. He got everything down in writing, then started the physical. Chest, back, stomach and knees. The lot. The way he went at the legs, I wouldn't have been surprised if they had come off in his hands. By the time he had finished I was more than a bit sore, and tender around the joints.

'Satisfied?' I asked him.

'Yes, I don't think there is much I don't know now, do you?' I shook my head.

'Nothing more today. The ward round is in the morning, and then you will see us all. After that, Tuesday is the big day. Be seeing you.' The book came out, and the time passed quickly by. Friendships were made, cards and dominoes played with the lads who couldn't get out of bed. This was a very important part of the ward life, helping the ones who were fastened to their beds for weeks and months at a time.

Monday morning, and all action. Now, a ward round in this hospital was really something. It was a military operation. Beds made, lockers dusted, patients practically sat up to attention in beds that were spotless, and as tidy as possible. The round looked more like a 'cooks tour' than anything else. There were more doctors and students than there were patients, or so it seemed to me. When they crowded round the patient's bed, whilst the surgeon described the ailment, and then the possible cure, they all seemed to surge to the front. The crunch came when he looked around for someone to do the same. For then, the back of the crowd seemed to be more popular than the front. My turn now, they were like flies near a jam pot.

'Good morning Mr Hill, how are you?' He might be the terror of the house doctors and students, but to me his bedside manner was a tremendous thing.

'Fine thanks.' You fool, I thought, you wouldn't be here if you were!

'Well tomorrow is the day, and I don't think we will disappoint you.' He then took his followers to the centre of the ward to examine my x-rays. Just before he eventually marched them all away, he came across and marked the knee with an arrow. They do this to make sure they operate on the right knee. He smiled and was gone.

Now it was action stations, the leg shave was expertly done, and then I had a bath. Twice during the day I had visits from the students to have a look at the knees. Each time I had to relate my history, still, I didn't mind if it helped them. The last thing that happened before the day staff departed was the clear out of the bowels. Yes, the insertion of the silver bullets. I had to suffer the same cheeky comments as the nurse rolled me over and saw my very hairy bum. Before she made the attempt at insertion, she stood up and had a look at the thinning hair on my head.

'Well?' I asked.

'Oh, I was just checking that I had the right end down here,' she said. Then she returned to her task, and succeeded at last. I steeled myself for about five minutes, and then I was off. On my return I was a very much lighter man, by a long chalk.

The orderly arrived with the milk drinks. I had my usual tea.

'That is your last, as you well know,' the nurse told me. The Sister arrived with the drugs. I accepted and swallowed my sleeping pill. In about two minutes flat, I was gone.

Dawn broke. From the noise, it broke into about a thousand pieces. I had thought that some of the other hospitals I had been in were noisy, but this one won hands down. Even the stuffing of my head under the pillow didn't help. A hefty belt on my backside made me sit up with a jerk. A washing bowl was thumped down on my locker and I was given about two inches of water for my ablutions.

'Can you spare it?' I asked, sticking my finger in. The water came to half way up my finger. The nurse swung the jug threateningly in my direction.

'Sorry!' I shouted, and ducked. I washed, shaved and preened myself, ready for the day's events. The time had raced by, it was now 6.10 a.m. Or the way they were dashing about, you would think it had.

'Is it always like this?' I asked my neighbour. Guess what I got in reply? Another grunt. 'A charming fellow,' I thought, 'his tongue must be in plaster. If it isn't, it should be.'

The nurse and her assisting orderly seemed to be doing all their chores at a dead run.

'If you two don't slow down and stop running round in circles, you are going to disappear to the place all such people go to, and are never seen again.' I was telling them this as they were making my bed. 'It is a bit of a bum joke that.' My words were wasted for they literally tore round the ward. 'What a life,' I thought, 'they must be crackers to do it.'

The day staff soon joined them, and breakfast was distributed. It smelt great and I was ravenous. It was really cruel, I thought, to dish it all out from the end of my bed.

'Any chance of a bit of a nibble Sister.'

Talk about put your foot in it. The wag up the ward who said, 'Before or after breakfast?' didn't help me much.

'Choose your words more carefully Mr Hill,' the voice was very stern. 'There are very young nurses on this ward.'

'You daft old bat,' I said to myself, 'these girls see men in the nude, wash them, shave them, everything. All there is to see on a man, they have seen.' But to please her, I smiled and said meekly, 'Sorry Sister.'

Everything was soon cleared away, then the day began in earnest. I watched carefully as the staff nurse wheeled the trolley into the ward. She slowly worked her way along the beds, aided by a young nurse preparing quite a number of patients for the theatre. It was obvious to me then that I was not going to be high up on the cutting list today. Eventually they reached me. Yes, I was the last one.

'It must be a good play today, for it seems as if everyone is going the theatre.' I wasn't very happy really, for it meant that I was going to have to lie there and think too long about what was going to happen. That didn't appeal to me one bit, nor did it appeal to my religious belief, that of a devout coward.

'Don't worry Mr Hill, the time soon passes, and you will have had an injection to calm your nerves.' This she told me as she shaved then painted away at the leg. It finished up a ghastly yellow colour. They wrapped it, and moved away to leave me to my thoughts. Don't worry, she said. How can you not worry at a time like this? I picked up a book and started to read. It was a waste of time, for I read the same line over and over again. So I lay there and watched, as in turn, the lads departed on the theatre trolley, through the door at the end of the ward. I just couldn't take my eyes off those doors as I waited for someone to return.

The clock ticked away, but not fast enough for me, then through the door the trolley returned bearing its victim back to his bed. The nurses crowded round and heaved him into it. I went white and felt sick. Oh no, I said to myself, don't be sick before you go this time as well. Two more returned in similar fashion before I saw the Sister walking towards my bed. I could see the needle on the dish she carried. Thank God, I whispered to myself, another expert, for I didn't feel a thing.

'It won't be long now. Just close your eyes and forget everything.' She smiled and left me.

They make me laugh, these people (even though I know they mean well), it is either 'be calm', 'now relax', or like now, 'forget it'. How in hell's name you can do that when you are lying there waiting to go into some unknown place for an operation, I'll never know. In my case it wasn't to be a huge operation, but brother, it was enough to scare me half to death. The theatre orderly arrived to transport me away. I slid across to his trolley from my bed.

'Away we go mate.' I tried to sound cheerful.

The journey was soon over, we even had a ride in a lift. As I waited to be put to sleep, the surgeon came over to see me.

'Good morning Mr Hill.' He was dressed in his green surgical overall, cap etc. and white rubber boots. I was to remember this very many times. I tried to smile up at him, it was a weak effort. Another needle in the back of my hand, the reverse count 'Ten, nine, eight, sev . . .' Oblivion.

There was the ceiling looking down at me. Both that and my head were spinning ever so slightly, but for all that, I didn't feel too bad. A bit sickly but not too much, that was good. And a fair amount of pain in the leg. Now that I was glad about, for I knew immediately that this time something had been done. As if to confirm my thoughts, suddenly, looking down at me was the surgeon.

'Well my lad, that should put that knee right.' He then smiled and left. Inside I felt great. At last I was going to be rid of the pain. I was sick for a while, but I didn't care half as much about that.

As time went by, the leg started to hurt a great deal.

'How are you feeling now Mr Hill?' It was Sister.

'Not bad thanks, although the leg hurts quite a bit,' I replied.

'I will be along soon to give you something to ease that.' She checked my pulse and temperature. 'Remember to drink plenty, it will help you with your waterworks.' She could rest assured on that, for I remembered only too well my last experience in that direction. Sister arrived again with her tray and needle.

'Roll over a little please.' It hurt the leg like hell to do just that. There was a rub of the thigh, and bingo! In goes another needle. After this I closed my eyes and gladly went to sleep.

It was only when I awoke, feeling much improved, that I dared to take a peep at the leg. Not knowing what to expect, I lifted the sheets. As there was a wire cage keeping the bedclothes away from my leg, I was able to see the full length of the bed. To say I was alarmed was a gross understatement; I was scared out of my very life. Starting at my thigh, then downwards towards my ankle were masses of bandages, the leg looked huge. I steeled myself and tried to move the thing. My God, nothing happened! I believed that they had put me right, but what had they done? It didn't bear thinking about. A most pleasant thing broke my thoughts, I found that I needed to use the bottle. I reached out and fumbled on my locker for one. As I reached over to my right, my weight moved my leg.

'Oh bloody hell!' I flopped back quickly, which had the same effect. The pain from my knee was excruciating. A nurse came over to me.

'Can I get you anything Mr Hill?'

'I want a bottle please nurse. I tried to reach my own but the stretching played havoc with the leg.' I used polite words for I saw Sister approaching.

'Trouble?' she asked.

'Not really Sister, it is just that I moved my leg. With rather unpleasant results.'

'Well you shouldn't, should you?' she said. The nurse explained that I had been reaching for the bottle.

'That's good, have you managed anything?' she asked. My reply was to produce, from under the sheets, the almost full bottle that I had been using whilst we had been talking.

'How's that then?' I asked proudly. She smiled briefly as she handed the bottle to the nurse.

Over the next couple of days I progressed quite well, and it was decided to transport me to the hospital's convalescent home. This was great for it was nearer home. The ambulance ride posed no problems, for I was feeling really good and on top of the world. I felt even better on my arrival, for the home wasn't really like a hospital at all. The ward was small and very light. But best of all, my companions for the next few days were a really pleasant bunch. To say that much of the time was spent in laughter is no exaggeration. Jokes flew about, fast and furious, clean, dirty, and even filthy.

The days raced by and then the big one – the removal of my great bandages, and the splint that went with them. My eyes were firmly fixed on the leg, for I really wanted to see what had been done. The staff nurse cut away the yards of bandages and padding, and then the splint.

'Hold that ton weight that you are always complaining

about,' she said as she passed it to me. I was flabbergasted. It was so light, it was only a metal alloy back splint.

'Bloody Nora, would you believe it!' I said.

'My name isn't Nora, and yes I would.' She removed the last piece of dressing. 'There it is, and it has healed perfectly, so I was wrong, there must be some good in you after all.' I stared at the knee. The scar was about ten inches or more long, and as I counted, I could see about twenty stitches.

'Wowee,' I hadn't expected anything quite like that. She gently cleaned the congealed blood off the stitches, and then started to lift and cut them away most carefully. I hardly felt a thing. A new dressing and it was all over.

'When can I go home?' I asked quickly. She laughed loudly.

'Not yet my lad. This bit has been easy, the physiotherapists want you next.'

'What do I want them for?' I demanded foolishly.

'To teach you how to bend your leg and walk again.' She packed her trolley.

'Rubbish!' I mumbled.

'Alright clever clogs, bend your knee carefully,' she told me.

'Right, I'll show you!' But I didn't. The movement I achieved was next to nothing. The pain I experienced whilst doing it, was just the opposite! 'My God, I don't believe it, all my life my legs have been the strongest part of my whole body. What the hell have they done wrong?' It was only then that I really took notice of my thigh muscles or quadriceps, and saw how distinctly thin and flabby they looked. There wasn't a sign of a bulging muscle there. Compared to my right leg, my left looked like a slice of streaky bacon.

'Don't worry Mr Hill, they will get all your muscles back,' she told me, as she put back the cage and made my bed.

'How in hell's name will they do that?' I demanded.

'Bloody hard work, both on your part and theirs,' she answered.

I saw the surgeon the following morning. He looked at the scar.

'Excellent, a perfect healing. Another two or three days then you can go home.' He placed his hand on my thigh muscles, and flopped them about. He looked at me, then turned to the physiotherapist who was with him. 'He is all yours now.' She noted my name in her book.

'I will be back later to see you, Mr Hill.'

As good as her word, she was. Only now there were two of them. They surrounded me with screens and stripped the bed again.

'Off with the pants Mr Hill,' said the senior physiotherapist. They both had tape measures at the ready.

'We want to measure your leg,' added the other girl.

'Cheeky! Are we having some kind of kinky competition, girls?' I asked them quietly.

'Don't be rude, and if we were, you would be well down the list,' they both retorted. That put me in my place, and no mistake. 'Now seriously Mr Hill, we have to measure your quadriceps on the bad leg, and compare them to your good one, then we know how much we have to regain to make you as good as new.' They then measured the floppy muscles. 'They really have gone quickly.'

'Why is that?' I asked, 'for my legs have always been my strength, and they have been very well developed since I was a kid.'

'That is really the reason. Well built-up quads will deteriorate much more rapidly than comparatively unused ones,' they told me.

'Come on then girls, let's get on with it then.' I was raring to go.

'Steady now, we have to take it slow and easy at first.' They tried to restrain my impetuosity, but I was stupid and wouldn't listen, so understandably, they gave it me the hard way! They got hold of my good leg and felt the muscles.

'Lift your foot up and tighten your leg muscles really firmly.' I did so easily, and they really bulged. I felt quite proud as I looked at my leg.

70

'Good, now do the same with the other one,' they demanded. I tried, I really tried, but nothing happened. Absolutely nothing. There wasn't a ripple of a muscle, not even a flicker.

'Now do you see how much work we all have to do? And believe us, it is not going to be easy for you.' They had got through to me now.

'Sorry, I understand. What do you want me to do?' I was really determined.

'To start with, you have to keep trying, every five minutes or so, to tense your quads. Lift your toes, and really pull. And for the time being, that is all. But do it religiously.'

'Right, watch this,' I said. I pulled my toes upright, then really tried to tense my muscles, but there was no response. I heaved and strained, but still nothing.

'Try it with both legs,' the head physiotherapist told me.

'Right, watch this time.' I was determined. I forced both heels into the bed, toes erect, and pulled like mad. Success! My right leg bulged mightily, and my left gave the slightest of flickers. But at least there was definite movement in it. I tried again, and there it was again! I was dead proud.

'How's that then?' I asked them both.

'Good, but you must keep at it. Five minutes every half hour or so.' They made my bed and moved on to other patients.

As true as my word, I worked away at my chores. I tensed and pulled every thirty minutes, for I was determined to get my thigh muscles back in trim. Even though I didn't actively take part in any sport any more, I was still very proud of my strong limbs. It became a consuming part of my day, I had no time for anything any more. Even when I read or listened to the radio, it was constantly, pull up, press down, and tighten. On and on it went.

The following morning, the physiotherapist returned. She stripped off the sheets and cage.

'Have you been practising?' she asked.

'Just you hold those toes,' I told her. She complied with my request. I forced the back of my knee down on the bed, and pulled really tight. The movement wasn't all that much, but I had worked hard at it, and she knew I had. I could tell that in her face.

'Very good Mr Hill, very good.' She then moved from the end to the side of the bed. 'Now I want you to do the same thing, but this time I want you to lift your leg off the bed slowly.'

'Right' I said. I did everything fine, up to the lifting of the leg. There was nothing. No upward movement, nothing! I tried again, but got the same result.

'I told you it wasn't going to be easy, didn't I?' She smiled at me. 'Slide down the bed a little and try again.' I reached over my head, took a firm grip on the bed-head rail, and strained away. Once, twice, three and four times I tried. Then suddenly with an effort, I managed to lift the leg off the bed. Just an inch or two, but what a bloody effort. I was amazed, for it just about shattered me. I was soaked in sweat.

'Blimey! I just don't believe it, the stupid thing is as weak as water.'

'Keep trying like you are, and you will succeed in building it up again to its former strength.' She sounded convincing but I was not so sure. Seeing the doubt in my face she said, 'We can only show you what to do, and help you a little, but it is you, yourself on whom the real result lies, so keep trying Mr Hill.' To prove to her that I would, I lay back and had another go, and again managed to lift the leg another few inches.

'Good, keep on going at it. I will see you again tomorrow.' And away she went.

The rest of the day I exercised diligently, and by the end of it I could lift the leg a good foot off the bed. Also, I worked away at quad exercises, for I was absolutely determined to have my leg back to its former strength.

The next day I was allowed up. Previously, I had always been very keen to leap out of bed and be away. This time I was not so sure. Even with all my exercising, I was still only able to obtain a little flexion of my muscles in the thigh, and the whole leg still felt like a ton weight to lift. No matter how I strained and sweated, I still could barely lift the damn thing more than a few inches off the bed. The fact that the physiotherapist and nurse replaced the metal splint and securely strapped the leg from thigh to ankle, didn't add very much to my confidence in it being able to support my weight.

I needn't have worried though, for both the girls took good care of me. They swung my legs over the edge of the bed, helped me into my dressing-gown, and then stood me up.

'That's right. Up you get, and take all your weight on your good leg first.' I steadied myself with their aid. I felt a little strange, and I was reminded of pictures of cranes or flamingos that I had seen in the past. I imagined that I must have, to other watchers, looked very much like one of those birds.

'Thank you nurse,' the physiotherapist said. The nurse then left us to fend for ourselves.

My guide and mentor presented me with a walking stick (my first of many).

'Take this in your right hand and ease your weight ever so slightly.' She then explained carefully the art of leading with the good leg, then following through with the stick and bad leg, whilst the weight of the body was taken by the good one. After a few stumbling steps up and down the small ward, I got the hang of it, so we moved into the corridor and made for the stairs.

'Now it is the same principle going up, as walking. Good leg first, take the weight, then it is hand and rail, plus stick. Then follow through and up,' she explained carefully. We negotiated a few steps laboriously, but successfully.

'Good,' she said, 'now to descend. This time it is different. It is bad leg and stick in the left hand, down first. This supported by the right hand taking the weight on the rail, then follow through and down with the good leg. Try it in reverse and you will overbalance for sure.' I struggled for a few minutes, then succeeded in negotiating the downward steps. At the bottom I stopped, exhausted.

'Bloody hell, I am shattered.' I just couldn't believe it.

'Good lad, now you are ready for home,' she told me. As we made out way slowly back to the ward, she really drummed it into me that I must only remove the bandages and splint to exercise, and never try to bend it on my own. She needn't have worried, I was not that brave.

'What happens now?' I asked.

'Starting on Monday, you will come along to the hospital, to our physiotherapy department, three times a week for treatment.'

'I see,' I said, but I didn't. Not by the faintest stretch of the imagination did I know what lay ahead of me.

11

The following Monday morning saw me begin my first day as an out-patient. What was to happen this day was to be repeated almost ad infinitum over the next ten years.

I had been told to be prepared for the ambulance at about 8.45 a.m., so I was there on the dot, seated in my front room awaiting its arrival. The yellow vehicle eventually turned up an hour later.

'Good morning,' I said cheerfully, as I entered and took my seat. My greeting was returned in the same manner, by the two elderly lady passengers already inside. I looked at my watch. My appointment was for 10 o'clock, so as it was almost that now, I asked the driver if we would be going straight to my destination.

'Heck no, lad! I have three more pick-ups yet, and then three hospitals to call at before yours, so settle down and make yourself comfortable, for you will be with me quite some time.' So began my first 'ambulance mystery tour'. We made our other collections and then visited most of the hospitals on the way into the city. It was a varied collection, a baby hospital, a cancer hospital, a foot hospital, then finally mine, a general hospital. There wasn't much, I was to find out by talking to people over the years, that couldn't be diagnosed and cured by some specialist in this place. There were obviously some exceptions.

The journey had taken about seventy minutes. Being my first visit, I was worried about being late.

'Don't worry lad, they won't expect you on time with us,' my driver told me. 'I will pick you up later today, in here,' he pointed around the room we had just entered. It was the transport department of the hospital. In this room, all the out-patients gathered after treatment, to be returned home to all parts of Manchester and its suburbs, by ambulance and hospital cars. It was an operation, in the main, organised by two ladies, who, as I was to appreciate over the years, did it really well. In addition, they did it, at the same time, most cheerfully.

Making my way to the physiotherapy department, I wondered what lay in store for me. The leg was quite sore as I limped along, and I wasn't very happy at all. I passed the x-ray department, and reached the stairs leading up to the department I was heading for. As I made my way up a step at a time, I was passed by some of the most beautiful girls I had ever seen. There seemed to be girls of every nationality and colour, there were blondes, brunettes and redheads. There were white girls, black girls, brown girls and yellow girls. As if some dowdy old lady had tried to distract men from seeing this obvious beauty, most of these girls wore a uniform that resembled that of an overgrown brownie. That it didn't succeed in doing so, was to the credit of the girls themselves.

I reached my floor and handed in my card to the office.

'Take a seat Mr Hill,' I was told. My name was soon called, and a small dark girl took me into a large room, which I was to share with numerous other patients. She led me to a vacant plinth and handed me a pair of shorts.

'Please remove your trousers, shoes and socks, and then put these on,' she told me. I did as requested and swung myself onto the couch. She returned with another lady, not in brown, but in white, and obviously in charge.

'Good morning Mr Hill,' she said. She then took off the bandage and splint. They measured both legs, asked me to tighten my muscles a few times, then lift once or twice. I did the best I could for them, but it wasn't very good, for I seemed to have deteriorated over the weekend.

'We have a lot of work to do here Mr Hill, and we can only help you if you want to help yourself.'

'You name it and I will do it,' I promised her.

'Good. Well he's all yours now,' she said, turning to the young physiotherapist. So the battle commenced in earnest.

The first minutes were spent in the quads, tightening and lifting the leg. It seemed even harder than in the hospital. I then rested a while and started over again. This went on for over thirty minutes.

'Good. Now before you go, we are going to try a little bending of the knee.'

'Oh no!' I gasped, for the knee seemed to be solid.

'Oh yes,' she said with a smile. She knelt beside the plinth, ready to measure the first bend. 'Ready?' she said, 'now try.' I didn't know what to expect, so I tried hard. I pulled my foot up towards my bottom, but not much happened. That is, apart from the pain. It hurt, but I laughed. For I was amazed. I had pulled, expecting my knee to bend. All right, even if I expected pain, I did think it would bend. But it certainly didn't.

'That isn't very good is it?' I said to her. She shook her head.

'No it isn't. Now try again.' I did, and this time I pulled harder still. It was painful, but at least I succeeded in a bend of a few degrees. She strapped my splint back on, and helped me on with my things, for the knee was by this time not at its best.

'Mr Hill I want you to really practice the quad exercises hard. The stronger they get, the sooner the knee will bend. Keep trying all the time.' I promised her I would, and I meant it.

'Goodbye, I will see you on Wednesday.' She walked with me to the bottom of the stairs. 'Very good.' Well that was something.

Making my way back to the transport room, I knew that I was going to have to work very hard at my exercises. I was determined. I handed my name in at the desk, and took a seat. It was just 12.30 p.m. The room was quite full. 'How long will I have to wait here?' I wondered.

It was just turned 2.00 p.m. when the driver who brought me in came through the door.

'Mr Hill, Sale,' he shouted. Up I got with an effort.

'That's me, mate,' I said.

'Away we go then.' He led me away. 'Never give us up 'til its gone seven!' he laughed. I quickly learnt to accept the hours spent waiting for these lads. It was a difficult job, and you usually had to wait until the same driver who delivered you to the hospital, was able to return and collect the same people. So you usually had the same long journey home, as you had when you arrived. It couldn't be helped, that I was sure of. I arrived home at 3.50 p.m. At least it is time-consuming, I thought to myself.

The first week passed quickly by, with my physiotherapist not pushing me too hard, but continuing to concentrate on the quad build-up, and just straight leg raising. I was just as keen at home, on the same exercises, and really tried concentrating on the build-up of my muscles. The second week was much different.

I had arrived at the department, and taken up my position on the couch. I was doing my leg raising while I waited for my young lady to finish with another patient. Up in the air I lifted the thing, and was busily swinging it from side to side when my little 'brownie' arrived.

'Very good Mr Hill, I can see that you have been hard at it over the weekend,' she said innocently.

'Hey, now then, don't be cheeky,' I said naughtily. She burst out laughing.

'I didn't mean that!' She took out her tape to check the thigh. 'Very good, but now we come to the hard part, and of course, that means knee bends, so here we go.' I swung my legs over the edge of the plinth, and sat with the good leg bent against the edge, and the other sticking out straight ahead – what is more, with not a sign of a bend anywhere near it. She gently took hold of the foot with one hand, and then placed the other just behind the knee.

'Ready now, here we go.' As she spoke, she gently put pressure on the foot. I helped as much as I could, by trying to force the leg to bend a little. Our combined efforts

78

achieved very little, so we tried again, with no success. The joint was as solid as a rock.

I was allowed to rest for a little while, then we started where we had left off, with the exercise again, over and over again. All to no avail.

After this I was allowed home, to return the following day. And it went like this, day after day. Each time a little bend, plus the sight of a little more muscle. Three weeks of individual treatment, and at last I could sit on the plinth with both knees almost perfectly bent, and then swing both legs up to almost level, out in front of me. I could repeat this three or four times before the left leg started to give me pain.

The following week, the departmental head examined me, and transferred me to what was known as the 'quads' class. I was to start the next day.

On my arrival at the department the following day, I was to find that I was just one of a crowd. There seemed to be dozens of us, limping along to get changed into our blue hospital shorts. We were an assorted lot, that's for sure. Short, tall and medium. Thin, fat, obese and normal. I prided myself that I was in the latter group. We were split into groups by three young physiotherapists. Whilst they looked terrific in their skin-tight trousers and yellow blouses, we, by comparison, must have looked a motley lot in our ill-fitting shorts.

Once they had sorted us out, they really went to town on us.

'Get those mats out gentlemen.' They pointed to a stack of thick mats that were in the corner of the gym. We spread them on the floor as instructed.

'All down on your backs, and legs out straight,' was the command. Down we eventually got, but some of us had a struggle doing it.

'Right legs, raise!'
'Right legs, lower, slowly!'
'Left legs, raise!'
'Left legs, lower!'

Then we had a change.

'Bad legs, raise.' A pause. 'Now swing to the left. Now to the right. Now down, slowly.' Moans and groans could be heard all round the room, as we lay back on the mats, exhausted.

'Now then, hands on hips, and force your legs up into the sky.' I didn't do too badly, but there were some that were having a struggle to keep their legs up.

'Now, cycle! Come on now, give those knees the full bend.' You must be bloody joking, I said to myself. Apart from the legs, I classed myself as in my prime, but I was really struggling, so I could understand the assorted grunts and wheezes that were being emitted around me. But we pedalled away, closely watched by the girls.

'You can rest for a minute or two now,' we were told.

'They are sodding sadists!' panted the man lying next to me. As I turned to look at him, I could see the mountain that was his belly, heaving up and down.

'Mats away please,' we were told next.

'Thank God for that,' I said to myself as I stood up.

'Now for the forms.' Now what were they up to? We carried the half dozen long forms from the back of the room and placed them in two rows facing each other. The girls taking my group divided us up into two teams. We then had to pass a ball with our feet, from one to the other, and see who could get the thing to the top of the row and back first. It sounds easy but it wasn't. You had to keep your legs very straight all the time. Another short rest.

'Now for the beans,' called the girl. 'Could it be food?' I thought. I should have known better. These beans were in small bags. The physiotherapist walked along, throwing a few at our feet until we were all armed and ready to go. The object of the exercise seemed to be the gathering of one of the bags between your feet, then hurling it at your opposite number on the other form.

Direction wise, few of the bags reached their target, but shot off in all kinds of way out places. Once I got the hang of it, my missiles were accurately aimed at my tormentor,

80

my physio. I never learn, and I should have known better than to tangle with authority. For as the end of the session was called for the day, the darling girl called me to one side. She backed away into the corner of the room, beckoning me with her finger as she moved back. I followed hesitantly, for I didn't like the look on her face. Then I saw it. A bicycle, a kind of bicycle on a stand.

'On you get,' she said, with mock sternness.

'What now?' I said, as I sat on my perch.

'Pedal!'

'Alright,' I said. Only it wasn't that simple. My left leg was down straight, whilst my right knee was bent, ready to push. So I pushed. As the right leg pressed down, the left started to bend a little. I stopped at once and stared at her. It was bloody murder!

'You must be joking, I can't do that,' I laughed at her.

'Oh yes you can, and you will. Come on, force the knee to bend.' She wasn't joking now. 'You must try harder.' I could see she was serious, so I started again. I forced with all my strength, and ever so slowly it started to bend. But it hurt like blazes, sweat dripped off my face and body. I pushed even harder, and little by little, the right foot went down and down. As it did, the left knee came up higher and higher, the more the bend, the more the pain. Perspiration rolled off me. My God it was hard work.

Success! The bend was achieved, but I was shattered, and sagged on the handlebars.

'Well done Mr Hill, that will do for today.' She helped me off the instrument of torture. I couldn't believe it, just one full turn of a bicycle pedal and I was exhausted. You would have thought to see me, that I had just participated in the annual Milk Race.

After I had changed, I staggered down to the transport room to wait for my ambulance, and home.

I continued to work away at the exercises at home. It would have been easy to give up and not to bother at all, but I thought the harder I pushed myself at home, the easier it would be for me at the hospital. In the physio department, the pressure was always on. We did all the exercises I had carried out on the previous visits there, but they could always come up with something new. Today was no exception.

The forms were out for we had been playing our simple ball games again. I was beginning to find that these were quite easy to do, so they didn't bother me at all. After she had collected the beanbags and plastic balls, the physiotherapist clapped her hands.

'Now gentlemen, I want you to stand in front of the forms like this.' She placed herself within stepping distance of the form. 'Then this is what I want you to do.' She stepped onto the form, leading with the left leg, and then she stepped down. Then she did the same leading with her right leg and down again.

'Ready, set, go!' she commanded. 'Up. Down. Up. Down.' We all stepped up and down for ages, she gave us no respite, on and on she drove us.

'Rest now.' The words were heaven sent. We flopped down wearily.

'Right, once more. Come on, jump to it!' She walked up and down the line like a prison warder. 'Right, rest.' Still there was no respite. 'Now I want you to space yourselves out, and straddle the form like this.' She bent down in front of me, with one leg either side of the form. She stretched down and gripped the form with both her hands. She was a beauty! As she bent down, her shapely behind in my face, my mind was far from thinking of straddling the form! I was quickly brought back to earth.

'Now all sit like this.' We all did. 'Bend your knees then push back, straightening your legs, again and again.' We did this time after time.

'Right, forms away, and that's all for today.' She released us with a smile.

I was on my way out when, 'Mr Hill, a couple of minutes on the bike please.'

'You must be pulling my leg,' I said. She shook her head and pointed to the corner, and I knew that she was not. I mounted the bloody contraption, and commenced to push down on the right pedal, at the same time gritting my teeth tightly. Up came the left knee, the higher the knee, the more the pain. In spite of that though, it was definitely improving. Over it went, then down and up we came again. Six times I did it, then my 'brownie' patted me on the back.

'Well done Mr Hill, that is enough for today.' I smiled my gratitude, and meandered away to change.

The time to meet the surgeon again had arrived, and as my progress in the department had gone from strength to strength, I felt that I must be ready for my discharge. The physiotherapy I now needed, I knew I could do myself at home.

I sat in the large hall waiting my turn to see the 'Chief', and as I sat there I was thinking to myself that it hadn't been too bad. Eight weeks had gone by since my operation, and the leg now felt really good. I had kept up with my exercises, and done plenty of walking, so the muscles were quite strong again. Also, my experience in the hospital, and the sight of other people suffering and in pain with much worse complaints than mine could ever be, had really enabled me to see my own trouble in its true perspective.

At last I was in with the surgeon. He examined the leg very carefully as I went through all the exercises.

'Very good. Well that is one done for you. We will leave it for a while and then send for you, to finish the other knee.'

'Thank you very much,' I said, shook his hand then left.

12

I had been discharged at the end of August 1964, and it was from then on that my nights were to be disturbed by a nightmare. It was the same practically every night.

In this strange dream I was back in hospital, in the same bed, and feeling very ill after an operation on my knee. As I lay there in great pain, I saw the ward doors thrown open, and in strode my surgeon. He was dressed in his theatre garb, his green clothes and white boots, his cap and his mask. And with him were his assistants. He approached the nurse by my bed.

'What seems to be the trouble nurse?' he demanded.

'The leg sir, it smells,' she replied. They whipped back the clothes and looked down at me.

'It will have to come off. Now!' the Surgeon said.

I always used to jerk awake at that same spot, absolutely and utterly terrified, and soaked in perspiration. This went on night after night. Though like a fool, I would tell no one about it, except of course my wife, Irene, for pyjamas had to be changed, and, at the worst, sheets also.

The weeks passed by, and then one day the phone rang at work. It was my wife to tell me that I was to go into hospital that coming Sunday. I looked at the calendar on my desk. It said Friday 13 November 1964. Superstition is, I know, stupid, but I wasn't very happy at the thought, especially with the combination of the date, and the damned nightmares. But in I went, though far from bravely.

For this visit, for a change, I went in the long side of the ward. I was very relieved for I had dreaded being given my old bed on the other side, for only the previous night I had dreamt my usual nightmare. The procedure prior to the operation was absolutely identical to my previous visit, with the one main disappointment; my surgeon was on holiday. Then the other senior consultant went down with flu. So I was in the hands of the chief registrar, he was going to carry out my operation. It didn't bother me overmuch, for they must all be good to work there.

The time came for me to go to theatre, and this time I was accompanied by a staff nurse from the ward, a very pleasant girl who lived close to me at home.

'Don't worry Raymond, everything will be fine.' We went to the anaesthetist's room where I had to wait for a little while. The surgeon entered and looked at both knees.

'Hello Mr Hill, I will try and make them a matching pair for you.' He smiled, and left me to the knockout doctor and my staff nurse.

'Well you know all about this by now, so I will go ahead and give you the injection. Just a gentle prick,' he said, and in it went. I lay there, he sat there, and the staff nurse stood looking down at me. We all looked from one to the other, for nothing was happening. I squeezed the hand of the nurse, 'I am still awake.' My mouth felt dry but that was all. Looking at the anaesthetist, I asked what was wrong.

'Are you a heavy drinker Mr Hill?'

'No, I only drink a little, if at all. Why, what is wrong?' I asked again.

'It is very strange, for this only happens to very heavy drinkers, but don't worry, I will have to give you another one.' I wasn't too happy, but there was nothing else for it. There was no going back.

This time I watched the needle go in, but I didn't see it come out. I went out like a light, no time to even count one.

My eyes opened, and I felt absolutely terrible. I was vomiting like I had never done before. One nurse was holding a bowl for me, and I was filling them in quick succession. My whole body was soaked in sweat, and I felt as though I was on fire. Then I noticed that the house doctor was also with me.

'You feel dreadful don't you Mr Hill? Never mind, it will soon wear off.' He was going to get no prizes for that observation, but at least he seemed very concerned.

The curtains were drawn around me so that my sickness wouldn't bother my neighbours, for I was heaving continuously. I vaguely remember seeing my wife at my bedside with the doctor, but she quickly left me to their care. I was given an injection, which quickly put me out. A long time later, I was awake again, not feeling very much better, but at least I felt part of the ward again. As I stirred I heard kind words flowing from my fellow patients in nearby beds. Then I heaved again, and their kind words changed to shouts of 'Nurse, a bowl, quick, for Raymond'. Not only the nurse arrived, the doctor also arrived at my bedside. I was glad, for I was still burning up.

'What's gone wrong, Doc?' I asked him weakly.

'You have a chest infection from the double dose of anaesthetic that we had to give you. The reason you are so hot is that your temperature is a hundred and four degrees,' he told me. I thought to myself, I knew I shouldn't have come this time, being sent for on Friday 13th should have warned me!

The following morning on the ward round I was very popular, for everyone gathered around me while my chest was sounded by first one and then the other. My chart also seemed to make very good reading for them all.

'How are you feeling this morning,' they asked, almost in unison. It was like a choir hitting their first note. What a bloody daft question, I thought to myself, for even as they pulled back the clothes to examine me, the steam from my hot body seemed to cloud up over them. Still, I suppose it was manners to ask. For all that, all I could manage in reply, was a very sickly smile.

I was glad when they all moved to the next bed and left me to be looked after by the very efficient ward staff. They were really doing a fine job to make me as comfortable as possible. I just wished the sickness would leave me for a while.

The next day was just the same, I still felt absolutely terrible, still hot and very sickly. On top of this I was sorry to say that the leg was really giving me some stick. I put this down to the fact that it felt worse because of my sickly condition, so consequently, I didn't complain about it when asked.

It was decided that as the ward was packed with accident cases, and more and more coming in all the time, I would be better off being shipped to the nice convalescent home. That was as soon as my temperature went down a few degrees. To await this, I was moved upstairs to another ward. This, as it turned out, was a surgical ward. Bladders, stomachs and the likes.

At first sight, I didn't like the looks of the place. It looked very old and antiquated, and everyone seemed to be old and very poorly. That I most likely looked the same didn't occur to me!

Two days passed, with no improvement in my condition. Quite the reverse, in fact. I felt ghastly, very hot, and the leg was giving me hell. The thing I couldn't understand was that I was lying there and not caring, but just seeming to resign myself to the condition I was in, and not complaining about my predicament to any of the new staff looking after me. Night came, and by this time I honestly didn't know where I was, for I was in so much pain. Fortunately for me, the young night nurse was very efficient. I was tossing and turning in the middle of the night, and now getting delirious.

'Mr Hill, can you hear me?' she gently whispered in my ear. I nodded, but I couldn't make out her face properly, everything was just a blur.

'Is it your leg or your chest?' she asked me quietly.

'My leg is killing me,' I told her through clenched teeth. She took the clothes off my bed cage, and felt my foot, and then examined it by the light of her torch. She covered the leg again, and shot out of the ward.

She was back very soon, with the night Sister, and my own house doctor. They quickly pulled the curtains around my bed and examined me. By this time I wasn't with them at all. That is until I felt the impact of a needle in my thigh, and even that didn't bother me much. Almost immediately, it was as if I climbed or floated out of my bed, and hovered there, looking at them and myself as they gathered around me. It was the strangest experience of my life, so strange and pain free, that I was convinced that I was dead. My body was suddenly cooled and felt no pain. Everything was peaceful. It was uncanny.

I awoke early the next morning to find myself still in bad trouble with my leg, and seemingly just as hot as ever. It was very disappointing, for my last recollection of my condition had been the one of peace and tranquillity from the previous night. Now here I was, just as bad as ever. What next, I wondered, and I thought how incredible that two very similar operations, for the identical complaint, could turn out to have such different results.

Suddenly, I was shattered and terrified. For through the door, came my surgeons, clad in their theatre clothes. The green garments, the white boots, the caps and the masks. Yes, the identical clothes of my nightmare. They approached my bed and removed the clothes and cage.

'I am sorry Mr Hill, but we will have to take you straight to theatre, while we have a look at this knee. This time there will be no anaesthetic for you.' He put his hand on my shoulder. 'Don't worry, it will soon be over.' If he but knew how terrified I was, for it was too much like my nightmare to be a coincidence. I knew I shouldn't have come into hospital this time, after being sent for on that dreaded date, Friday 13th.

The orderlies soon arrived for me, and I was quickly taken down to the theatre. There was no waiting for any injections this time, but for the first time I went through to the theatre wide-awake. I was lifted very gently off the trolley onto the operating table, under the giant lights. As I looked up, I could see my reflection in them. My leg was lifted gently by the Sister, while the bandages and then the splint, were removed. Then finally, the dressing over the wound was taken off. The knee was the size of a small football, and all discoloured and puffy. I was in intense pain now.

'Why didn't you tell us before, that your leg was as bad as this?' they asked me sharply.

'I was all mixed up, and I just thought that I had a more serious operation. Then after a while, I just thought it was all a part of my condition,' I told them. They redressed the wound, then replaced the splint and bandages.

'Oh, that feels better,' I said.

'I can believe that,' said a theatre nurse, as she wiped my wet brow, 'for with that swelling, the bandages had become far too tight.'

I was taken from the theatre, back to my own ward. Not only that, but I was put into a side ward where my bed end was tilted high in the air. I received another injection, and was left to lie quietly, until I drifted off to sleep. The combination of numerous injections, and a constant supply of brandy and milk over the next few days, helped my body temperature to get back to normal. The knee was still a very big problem, both in seriousness and size, for the pain was still my constant companion, and the swelling was showing absolutely no sign of leaving me. I was a problem.

Obvious dissension as to the method of treating the knee was also very much in evidence. There seemed to be two schools of thought on the subject. One taking the line that the badness and fluid should be drained, the other that it should be left as it was for a few more days. As this was the thought of the senior consultant, this was the line that was adopted, for the present at least.

I spent over a week in the side ward, lying there on my own, and I didn't like it one little bit. I was badly missing the comradeship of the other men in the ward. I was constantly begging the Sister to have me moved back, but she wouldn't. Or as she insisted, couldn't, not without the senior consultant's permission. So I was determined to ask him to have me moved as soon as I saw him again. My chance came when they decided to look at the knee once more to check on the infection.

The Sister herself came in to prepare me for my multitude of VIPs. She stripped off the bandages and removed the splint, then gently cleaned up the still very badly swollen knee. It looked a horrid and ugly mess. It was a myriad of colours, yellow, black, green and a dirty purple. When she had completed her task, she covered the wound with loose gauze dressing.

The sounds of numerous footsteps and hum of hushed conversation heralded the arrival of my visitors. They all followed the 'chief' into the small room, and soon there was room for no more. All were masked; even the ones that couldn't get in and were still out in the corridor. Sister removed the loose dressing from the knee so that they could all have a good view of the thing.

'Good morning Mr Hill, I hope you don't mind all these visitors. I will send them away if you do.' I shook my head and said that I had no objection. He put his hand on my forehead, then felt my pulse.

'The fire seems to have died down at last, doesn't it Sister? But unfortunately, this knee hasn't seemed to improve very much since I last looked at it.' He bent forward and gave the joint a really keen scrutiny. 'What do you think?' he asked, turning to some of his students. They queued up to take a peek, and then pass their opinions to him as to how to treat it. He listened to their words intently, but it was obvious that he had already decided what was going to happen to it. He beckoned the Sister and house doctor forward, and pointed to the eighteen or so black stitches that seemed barely to be holding the cut together.

'I want you to remove just two stitches a day, one from each end of the incision. Take them out with great care, and be sure that this leg is not allowed to bend an inch.' He turned and spoke to his audience; 'I am not prepared to drain the wound at this stage, as I think Mr Hill has been through enough for the time being.' I knew of one registrar for sure, who was dying to take away the mess that was there, for I had heard him discussing it with the staff nurse the previous day. Just as it seemed that they were about to leave me, I ventured to ask the great man the request that I had made earlier to the Sister.

'Can I ask a favour please?' I ventured.

'Yes certainly Mr Hill,' he said, 'what is it?'

'I want to go back into the big ward if possible please. I am not one for being on my own, I much prefer to be with the other lads.'

'If it's alright with Sister, then I certainly have no objections now.' Then off he went, his protégés trailing behind him. The staff nurse came in to help the Sister carefully replace the splint and bandages.

'Back in the long side with him after lunch please Staff, he has just pleaded his case successfully with the "big man". Though I think before we move him we will have him sat on a bedpan. I think it is about time his bowels were encouraged to move.'

'I don't feel as if I want to go on a pan yet Sister.' I hadn't been since having my operation. 'And I have been very good this time with my water works, and that is much more important, or so everyone tells me.' I really didn't want them to manhandle me on to the damn thing. I had to work hard to convince her, but I am glad to say, I won.

'We will leave it then, but I am going to give you some really good laxative the next time I come round with the medicine trolley.' She made it sound more like a threat than a promise.

A little time later, I was wheeled into the long side, to the very welcoming cheer of my friends. It was great to be back with them. I was visited by all the 'walking wounded' and we chatted away for hours. Conversation with my fellow bedfast friends was of the megaphone variety, but Sister soon came along and put a stop to that.

'Be quiet all of you, it sounds like a taproom in here. And you, Mr Hill will find yourself back in that little room very quickly. So less noise all of you.' My word, she did sound touchy, but we all realised it was for our own good.

It was afterwards that I started to feel the pain in my stomach, very faintly at first, but then as time passed by, it became much more severe. So much so, that by the time the evening visitors went, I was dripping with sweat yet again. I was rolling about, feeling sorry for myself, when the staff nurse came across to me.

'What is it Raymond, pain in the knee?' she asked. I shook my head.

'No, it is pains in the stomach.' She looked at my chart.

'You haven't had your bowels moved yet, have you?'

Shaking my head, I told her, 'I had some laxative this morning but nothing has stirred yet.'

'You are a troublesome patient you know. Do you feel as if you want to go or not?' She was asking this as she felt all around my stomach.

'No I don't. I have had hardly anything to eat since I came in here, and if there is nothing going in one end, I fail to see how anything can come out of the other. Do you?' It seemed logical to me if not to her.

'What about wind?' she asked suddenly.

'Well I know it's good for sailing ships.' It was asking for trouble, but I couldn't resist it. I looked at the raised arm fearfully, and cowered away.

'I mean are you breaking wind or not?' she demanded.

'No, not even the tiniest puff.' I told her. Away she went to quickly return with two manurish looking tablets.

'Take these and drink plenty of water. Lots and lots of it.' Then off she went for the day.

The combination of the pain in both the knee and now the stomach, didn't help me pass a very good night. So I was really glad when daylight came, for there is nothing worse, I think, than to spend a long sleepless night in a hospital ward. The only thing that enables you to come through many of them sanely, are the numerous cups of tea that devoted night staff constantly bring to you. All part of the tender loving care.

All the tea and water I drank certainly kept my bottle filling going to the maximum, but it did nothing for my pain-filled bowels. The arrival of the day Sister on the ward was soon going to put an end to my trouble, but I didn't know that when she came over to examine me. She drew the curtains around us, removed the bedclothes, and the cage, and said to me, 'Now, before we look at this knee and decide which stitches to remove, we are going to get rid of your troublesome "belly warts"!'

'Bloody great news! I think I would even look forward to an enema if I thought it would do the trick.' I was surprised at myself, but I meant it.

'You are not having one of those, but something very near it,' she told me. 'Ah here comes Staff to help me. The curtains were parted, and the trolley came through, propelled by the staff nurse. I quickly weighed up the contents on it, to see what fearful instruments it contained for them to use in their attempt to free me of my pain. All I could see was a bowl of water, and a length of rubber tube, plus a couple of rubber gloves.

'Now what?' I asked, as they pulled on the gloves. Sister lifted the tube. On one end was what appeared to be some kind of fitting.

'This end I have to screw gently up your bum, and the other end we place in the bowl of water. We will all know when we have succeeded, for the freed wind should cause some rather large waves in the water.' I just couldn't believe it was true.

'You're pulling my leg aren't you?' I laughed. That wasn't for long, for I saw that they were deadly serious. 'Oh no!' I exclaimed, and came over very sickly.

The staff nurse moved to one side of the bed and helped me to roll over towards her. It took a while with the leg being in the state it was. Then at last they had me poised for the kill. The Sister removed my fig leaf, and gently eased the cheeks of my hairy bottom apart. She bent down and forward.

'Ready Raymond, here we go.' She pushed and screwed, gently but firmly, that bloody horrible tube up my backside. Both the tube and my rear were liberally greased! I cringed and pulled my face, for it was agonising. Suddenly it hurt, and I went very tense.

93

'Sorry, I am being as gentle as I can. It won't be long now.' She sounded sincere. By this time sweat was pouring off me, for it was far from pleasant, and what was more, it was very humiliating. Or at least I thought it was. I was gripping the staff nurse's arm in a steely grip. I must have been hurting her but she smiled down at me kindly.

'Not long now,' she said.

She was right, for without warning the water in the bowl started to boil and bubble madly. It only seemed to last a few seconds, but the actual relief was immediate. All the pain and discomfort disappeared at once. It was fantastic, if I had been able to, I would have jumped for joy. Only the smell was odious! The tube was removed gently, like a cork from a bottle.

'Success for all of us. I'll bet you feel a hundred times better for that.' They eased me very carefully on my back again. It felt marvellous; I rubbed my hands over my stomach and felt nothing.

'I wouldn't have believed it possible, thanks very much to both of you.' I was overjoyed. It wasn't to last though, for the next words took my new found joy away.

'We will leave the curtains and come back at once to look at the knee.' And off they went, trolley and all.

As I lay there looking at the mountain of bandages that covered the leg, I wondered what it would look like now. Would the swelling have gone down at all. I was soon to know, for the Sister and staff nurse returned to me promptly. Between them they soon had the bandages and splint off. Whenever that happened there was a blind panic inside me! Even the slight movement of the leg as they removed the support, was enough to send searing pains shooting both up and down the leg.

It still looked a very ugly sight, swollen and discoloured, and the stitches still seemed stretched to the limit. It was as though the cut was just ready to burst open. It was a mess!

They were both masked now as they peered at it prior to the removal of the two stitches as instructed. The staff nurse bathed and cleaned the two stitches at the extreme ends of the cut, and the Sister then very carefully extracted these. As the stitches came away, some of the foul mess that was causing the swelling oozed its way through the holes. This was quickly and efficiently cleaned up, and the leg redressed. For this I was grateful, for I was a lot happier when I knew that I couldn't bend it, even the merest fraction. The last thing I wanted to do was to bend the thing, either intentionally or accidentally. They pulled the curtains, and I didn't feel too badly, for at least I had got rid of the wind, and as far as I was concerned, that was good enough for me. I didn't relish the idea of having to perch myself on a bedpan and commune with nature.

I settled myself down and read my paper, or tried to, for I had no sooner devoured the sports page, before I had another visitor. It was a vision in white, a physiotherapist.

'Mr Hill?' she enquired.

'Oh bloody Nora, now what?' But I already knew the answer to my own question.

'I have come to look at your left leg I think?' she looked at the pink card in her hand. 'Yes, the left one.'

'Well you can be very sure that you are not going to touch the right one, I can tell you that!'

'Now, now, don't let us get off to a bad start, we have to work in unison or we won't get anywhere.' She drew the curtains and rolled down my bedclothes, then gently lifted off the cage.

'Well I am willing if you are, though it could prove a bit tricky.' Oh dear, I thought, I hope she can take a joke. I needn't have worried, for not only was she very capable and efficient at her profession, but she was also blessed with a great sense of humour.

'Sorry Mr Hill, the only thing it tells me to develop, here on your card, are your quadriceps. Anything else is out.'

'Ah well, such is life, win a few, lose a few.' We had a good laugh, and at that moment, I felt better than at any time since my operation. What tremendously powerful medicine laughter is.

'Talking about quads, where are they, and what are these

things?' She was slapping gently at my muscles in my left thigh. 'You haven't been doing your exercises have you?'

'You must be joking, I have had to get help to open my eyes, let alone tighten my leg muscles. You may not know it, but I have been proper poorly, I have really.' I lay back and performed my 'dying swan' act again. She stood there for a moment and played an imaginary violin, but not for long.

'Seriously Mr Hill, you must work hard to build this leg up to its former glory. It is essential, for it has got a tremendous lot of hard work ahead of it.' I realised that what she said was true, the longer I stayed in bed, the worse and weaker the leg would become.

'OK lady, let's go. I am all yours to do with as you please.' And I was, she really put me through it. It was 'tighten, rest, tighten, rest'. Then again and again, and yet a few times more. This was then followed by a hard and tiring session of leg raising which seemed to go on and on. By the time she remade my bed and made me comfortable, I was well and truly shattered. If ever the saying 'cruel to be kind' applied to any profession, it certainly did to physiotherapy.

'I will be back in the morning for another session. Until then, I want you to really go to town on these exercises. If you don't, your leg will just fold up completely when you eventually get out of bed.'

'Cross my heart dear, I will put all my efforts into it, and that I really do promise.' I did too. Every spare minute I tightened and pulled away at my muscles, for I was determined to succeed and get back on my feet again.

Later in the day I began to feel the need of something that I had managed to do without so far in my stay in the hospital. Yes, it was a bedpan.

'Nurse,' I called over to one of the young nurses on the ward, 'can I try a bedpan please?' I wasn't keen on the idea, but I knew it had to be.

'OK Raymond, I will get some help, it could be a bit tricky.' And off she went, to return with a small army of helpers. There was the staff nurse, two other nurses, plus the ward orderly, and he was carrying a monkey pole. This was my first introduction to this most important piece of orthopaedic apparatus, which he soon fitted to the back of the bed. It was a curved bar that slotted into brackets at the head of the bed. Then it came up and over the bed in a curve. From it, was suspended a chain and a double hand-grip. Monkey poles, I was going to learn, were an invaluable part of my future hospital life, for the amount of relief to the cheeks of your bottom as you hoisted yourself up on the handle for a few seconds, was almost indescribable.

The small group surrounded the bed and prepared for action, with the staff nurse directing the operation.

'Now I want you to reach up and grab the handle, then, when I tell you to heave, I want you to take as much weight as you can so we can slide the pan under you. Right?' I nodded, and reached upwards and gripped the swinging handle as firmly as I could. The orderly and one of the nurses faced each other across the bed at my back. They joined hands to support me as well. The staff nurse unveiled the pan.

'Ready. Heave away,' she commanded. Up I went, quite well.

'Now down, gently,' she said. I lay there, half-swinging, half-leaning backwards on the supporting hands and arms and perched very precariously and uncomfortably on the damned hard pan. What is more, the top of the metal splint was caught on the edge of the bloody thing. I looked imploringly at them all as I half-lay and half-sat there, not at all happy, and decidedly not settled enough to perform as I thought I wanted to.

'You're joking aren't you, I can't manage anything suspended here like this, and with an audience. Help me into a more comfortable position, and then you can leave me for a while.' They all laughed at me but I didn't care. I wasn't bothered either that I was half-lying there in only my pyjama jacket, and even that was wide open, leaving me practically swinging there over the bedpan in a semi-horizontal and nude condition. I took a firmer grip on my pole,

97

and each of my helpers seemed to grab a different part of me, and between us, we managed to force my body into something more like a sitting position. I felt sure that by hanging on tightly I would be able to manage what by this time, I was desperately dying to do.

'Off you all go, I will be fine now. I will shout out loud if I need you.'

'Right then, we will, but be careful and lie still. Don't try to clean yourself up when you have finished, just leave that to us.' She looked at me carefully, and asked 'Are you sure you will be OK?' I nodded my head vigorously.

I sat there, or should I say swung there, in the most precarious position you could imagine, and then, with lots of effort, proceeded to empty my inner self into the bedpan. Whoosh! That part was over in seconds. Now, my original thought had been to wipe my own backside, clean myself, and remove the bloody horrible thing I was perched upon. All this mind you, whilst hanging from my monkey pole with one hand. Who was I kidding, by the time I had completed the first part of my task, that of filling the bloody pan, I was absolutely knackered! I was completely exhausted, I needed help, and I needed it quickly.

'Staff, in here please.' It was indeed a very plaintive plea. In a flash they were all back inside the curtains. I could only assume that they had been poised, waiting for such a cry of distress. They quickly sorted me out. They wiped me, washed and powdered me all over, remade my bed, and left me a much relieved and comfortable patient. T.L.C., thank heaven for the nursing service.

Now I may have been happier, but my friends and neighbours were definitely not, for scent sprays were working overtime.

'You stink awful, you must have been rotten inside.' Their cries were accompanied by more and more spraying in my direction. Suddenly, Sister appeared, a royal blue sergeant major.

'What is all this noise, remember people are sick in here.' I got the evil eye, then she was gone. But so was the noise!

The following morning was all hustle and bustle, in preparation for the consultant's round. Clean floors, tidy lockers and beds. Move if you dared when the beds had been made! As for myself, I was encircled by my curtains like some dusky Arab virgin awaiting a handsome Sheikh to ride up and take her all. My bed was stripped, and my cage, splint and dressing had been removed, and the wound was just covered with a piece of lint. I had also been given a clean fig leaf. The nurse had helped with the removal of the old one, and the replacement of the new. We were certain that if we had dropped the old one on the floor, it would have found its own way to the laundry basket. From my secluded spot, I could hear the large group moving around the ward, and then it was my turn. All we needed was a fanfare of trumpets!

'Let us see him Sister,' said the voice. Then I was surrounded by the pack. You could see the keen housemen or women pushing to the front, or the uncertain ones edging to the back of the group.

'Good morning Mr Hill, how are you today?' the great man asked. Before I could answer, he did it for me. 'Oh dear me, there doesn't seem to be much improvement there, but don't worry though, time will heal.' He looked at my chart. 'Continue with the antibiotics Sister, and continue with the slow removal of the stitches.' They all moved away, all bar one registrar. He was really weighing up the ugly and discoloured puffy mess that was my knee joint. Our eyes met over his mask, and I wondered if he felt that it should be attacked another way. He eventually followed the others with a brusque 'good morning'.

'I won't be a few minutes Raymond,' this was the staff nurse, 'then I will whip out another couple of stitches for you.'

'Gee thanks Staff, I can hardly wait,' I chided her. As good as her word, she returned with her trolley, and did the deed as kindly and efficiently as she could. But the removal of each stitch led to more pain, and more oozing of the messy substance that was inside the knee.

'It's a bloody horrible mess isn't it?' I was fed up with the situation, and obviously sounded it.

'Now, now Raymond, don't get disheartened. Just look around you and you will see lots of men worse off than you.' She was right.

'Sorry Staff, no more complaints from me,' I said.

My day was only disturbed by the visit from my physiotherapist, but even this was a pretty fruitless one, for as hard as we both tried, we could only infuse the very faintest of flickers of movement in the quadriceps. I was fed up, and there was very little flicker in me either.

The following morning in the midst of all the ward activity, I had a visitor. He arrived with perfect timing, just as the staff nurse arrived with the trolley to clean up the knee a bit prior to removing two more stitches. It was the registrar.

'Good morning Mr Hill,' he said, as he donned a mask. They both carefully swabbed the knee, and even as gentle as they were, every touch seemed just like a hammer blow. Then the doctor placed his hands gently under the leg, one beneath the joint, the other near the calf. I looked up at him, horrified! The knee had not been bent more than a fraction of an inch since the operation.

'Gently does it,' he said, as he eased the joint ever so very slowly. I grabbed for my monkey pole and squeezed like mad. The pain was tremendous, and in seconds I was soaking in sweat, half through pain, half through fear. He didn't bend it more than two inches or so, but the immediate effect was as if someone was stamping on my knee in hobnailed boots. Every stitch seemed to be trying to surpass the other with its pain output.

'This is bloody ridiculous,' he muttered.

'Amen to that,' I said through my gritted teeth.

'Shall I take the stitches out now?' asked the nurse.

'No, I will,' he replied, 'hang on to the pole,' he commanded. I didn't need telling twice, I was already hanging on for dear life, but I surely gripped even harder. I stared in disbelief as he laid hold of a stitch with a pair of tweezers, and gave a short sharp tug.

'Bloody Nora!' I yelled. Yet as I shouted, the sight of all the oozing mess coming out of the hole dispelled the sensation of the pain! My God, I thought to myself, what has he done. Though as he removed his mask, he looked quite pleased with himself. He gave me a smile and a wink and left without a word.

The staff nurse busily cleaned up the mess, redressed the leg, made me comfortable and was about to leave when the Sister appeared.

'I understand that the wound has aspirated itself Staff,' she said. 'When the stitches were being taken out I believe.'

'Yes the registrar was removing them for me when it happened.' She looked hard at me.

'Oh dear Staff, that doesn't sound right, he never touched you,' I said in my cheekiest voice.

'The stitches I mean Mr Hill.' She sounded very indignant a turned a very bright pink.

'Sorry Staff, I was only joking,' I said.

'Well now at least we can find out what has been causing all the trouble in that knee for you,' the Sister said. As they pulled back the curtains and left me, I felt curiously much improved.

The rest of the morning passed quickly, and with the arrival of lunchtime, I really felt ready for a meal for the first time since my operation. I did my dinner full justice, much to the pleasure of the Sister.

My physiotherapist arrived for my daily session, and it was only when she rolled back the sheets that I realised, and we both saw, that the bandages were soaked in blood. Boy, was I scared, I must have turned green at once.

'Don't worry, I will get help.' And she was gone. The Sister, staff nurse and the physiotherapist were back in a flash, and in no time at all they had all the bandages and splint removed. We all stared at the new knee that was there to behold, for most of the puffiness had gone, and although all the discoloration was still there, it looked 100

101

per cent improved from just a few short hours earlier. I just couldn't believe it.

'Look at that Sister, doesn't it look great?' I was fairly bouncing up and down with excitement.

'Now then Raymond, take it easy and don't get too hysterical. Even as good as it looks, you have a long way to go yet, so calm down.' They all decided that under the circumstances, there would be no exercises today. I think that for the first time, I was disappointed.

So for the next few days, it was exercises every hour on the hour. I would roll back the clothes and go to work. Rigorous exercises on my left leg, tighten, relax, over and over again. Then leg raising and bending, really giving it all I could. I knew that this leg had some hard support work ahead of it. With the right one it was a different story. By this time all the stitches had been removed, and the knee certainly looked something more like normal. All right, that was somewhat of an exaggeration, but things were definitely looking up.

The moment of truth was yet to come, for so far, all we had been doing had been simple quads exercises, but no bending. Then came the morning and I received not one, but two physios, and as they pulled the curtains around us I said, 'Oh what have I done to deserve this special honour?' Then at once I realised why! 'Oh no you wouldn't, not yet surely?' But I was very wrong, they would. Undeterred by my pleas, they rolled back the clothes, removed the cage, and started to work on the left leg. Both they and I were very pleased with the response. They then turned their whole attention to the still very painful right one. At first they just had me tightening my quads, or what there was of them. It was all very gentle. After a few minutes of this, I knew what was going to be next – leg raising, or shall we say attempting it. I remembered how I had been surprised by the lightness of the 'Thompson' alloy splint the last time, so I was prepared for a nice easy lift. It was now about three weeks since my operation.

'Now Raymond, gently ease your leg up off the bed.'

This, as she put her hands very gently under the bottom of my leg. As I pulled up my toes and pressed my knee down ready for the lift, I experienced a fair amount of pain but tried to ignore it and lift. Nothing happened. Absolutely bloody nothing. I tried again, harder, but still nothing happened. I felt devastated.

'Let's ease you down the bed a little more Raymond,' they said. This we managed all right, and this time I put my hands over my head and held on firmly to the headrail of the bed.

'Right, now try again.' One girl gently held down my left leg whilst the other one placed her hands again under the right one.

'Now then, here we go.' I lay there; my gaze firmly fixed on the light above my head as I very gently heaved away. The sweat trickled from under my arms, and also dripped from my forehead, but ever so slowly I managed to lift the leg just a few inches. I tried to hold it but it was useless, if it hadn't been for the young lass, it would have dropped the short distance hard, but she took the weight and gently lowered it to the bed.

'Good, now just once more,' she said. Up it went, easier this time, but I still couldn't hold it there myself. I was absolutely cream crackered.

'That will do for today. Now, I want you to do these exercises every hour at least, and five minutes for each leg. Do both legs at the same time, you will find it is easier that way.' Then off they went.

I hadn't achieved much I thought to myself, but at least they seemed to be satisfied. At least that must mean I had made some progress, because these girls, for your own good, are hard taskmasters. From then on, all my waking hours were devoted to these exercises, for I was determined to be out of bed as soon as I could. Christmas was only three weeks away, and I was longing to be home by then.

The following morning, I was visited by the consultant and his followers, and was closely examined again.

'Well Mr Hill, we have found out what caused your

infection. It was thrush and this is a complaint that is usually associated with pregnant women.' He smiled and said, 'There was enough yeast in your knee for you to have started your own brewery.' At least he seemed glad that it was nothing more serious, so that made two of us that were happy in that respect. Then he had to spoil it didn't he. He felt around the quads and calf muscles, then turned to the Head of the Physiotherapy Department.

'There is a hell of a lot of work to be done here yet. What about the bending?' Oh no, I groaned inwardly, what did he have to bring that up for?

'We haven't started yet,' she replied.

'Well do so, but don't press him too hard just yet.' He patted my feet and led everyone away.

I lay there thinking about commencing the bending of the knee. I didn't fancy that at all, I remembered all too well, the problems we had with the left leg.

Time went by quickly until the arrival of my physiotherapist. She stood looking at me from the end of the bed.

'I believe you have had your visitors this morning, so now you know what to expect.' Rolling back the bedclothes, she said, 'Well let the battle commence.'

Soon she had the leg bared for action. First of all we went through the quads build-up exercises. Toes up, tighten up. Press the knee down hard as I could into the bed. Then it was Press! Press! Press! Now relax! Tighten! Relax! Tighten! She rapped these commands for a good ten minutes.

'Now rest a while.' That was the nicest thing anybody had said to me that day. I was under no illusion though. It would only be for a short time, that was for sure.

'Now then, here we go. Leg raising first.' She said this as she gently slid one hand under my knee. I was grateful for that.

'Ready, toes up and pull tight. Now come on, lift.' It was an effort, but I did it first time. Only about six inches, but more important was the fact that I was able to hold for a few seconds, then lower it myself. Wowee! She was more pleased than I was.

'Great Raymond, really great.' She was all smiles. 'Did you notice your quads starting to work. It is very obvious that you have been doing your homework. We can only help you if you help us.' How right she was. We repeated the leg raising procedure three more times, and each time I did it, I really seemed to be getting much more control of the lift. It was still hard and took great effort, but now I knew I was winning! I was soon brought down from cloud nine and back to reality.

'Do you want a drink before we start again?' I was wiping my face with a damp cloth to remove the moisture on my face. I needn't have bothered. I reached over to my locker to pour myself a drink, but before I could reach it she had done it for me. It somehow seemed to me that she was trying to delay the next stage of events.

'I don't know who is more scared of what's next, you or me. Don't worry, it's *my* knee.'

This was stupid, me trying to console a physiotherapist, but it did the trick, for she immediately said, 'Right, let's get at it then.' Within seconds, I knew why she was reluctant to start on me. She had eased one hand under the knee, and one gently on my foot.

'Now try to ease your foot gently up the bed, but go very steady.'

The very first movement was enough to let me know the reason for the lady's reluctance. It was sheer agony. The foot didn't make much progress up the bed, but every minute fraction of movement was purgatory. Bravery I had always been a little short on, so I cried out, 'Bloody Hell! This can't be right.' Though I did at least try to continue the movement.

'Stop now!' she cried, 'don't do it any more.' I didn't need telling twice, and I couldn't have moved it any more anyway, because it was now stuck solid. All we had achieved was just enough bend for her to move her hand upright under the knee, about four inches at the most. All that toil,

105

sweat and pain just for that. To me that didn't seem progress at all. No way!

'Now ease it down very carefully.' From her tone of voice she seemed pleased. Either that, or relieved, I wasn't sure which, and I wasn't going to ask. Slowly I eased the leg down and found that that was also extremely painful, but nowhere near as bad as going the other way. What a blessed relief when it was over. My respite was short lived.

'Let us try again Raymond, we have no secrets from each other now, have we?' At least she sounded sincere.

We tried as before, with gentle movements up the bed, but with a little more pressure from her and a little more effort from me. The harder we both tried, the worse the pain.

'I don't think I can stand much of that, love, I'm sorry.' I didn't want to sound frightened, but I was. The waves of pain were shooting up and down my leg. It was sickening!

'OK Raymond, that will do for now. Enough is enough,' she said. I could have kissed her for those few words. She quickly re-bandaged me up, nice and securely. What a blessed relief to feel the safety of the splint once more. Anyway, one thing was for sure; I felt I knew all that was ahead of me now. If only I had realised how wrong I was, and what the future would hold for me, I don't know what I would have done.

As it was, the days went by with, as hard as we tried, little or no more bend in the knee at all. The only progress we seemed to be making after hour after hour of hard physiotherapy, was that my quadriceps in both legs seemed to be getting stronger. I was beginning to think that I would end up with a permanently stiff leg. I was even more convinced of this when I was told I would be going home the day before Christmas, after a stay of about six weeks or so.

The leg was still supported with a splint, and tightly wrapped, so on the morning that I was due to go home, my physiotherapist arrived at my bed with a pair of crutches. My first ones! With the help of a nurse, she perched me on

106

the side of the bed whilst I put on my dressing-gown and slippers. Then came the big moment.

'On your feet Raymond, and take all your weight on your good leg.' This she said with a wry smile. 'Then take all your weight from your leg to your arms on the crutches, making sure to support yourself from the handgrip, and not letting the crutches rest under the armpits.' She made it all sound so simple. Eventually I was stood upright.

'Now steady yourself and get the feel of them before you attempt to move at all,' she told me. She needn't have bothered, for I certainly wasn't going to move. I went to sit back down again, but this move was quickly foiled.

'Oh no you don't!' and I was pulled back into an upright position.

'We are going to the top of the ward and back, and that's for sure.' She was very firm now. 'So off we go!' They practically frog-marched me there and back, and happily for me, straight into the arms of the ambulance men.

Home for Christmas! Brilliant! 1964.

13

I had a few days rest over the festive season, as most of the physiotherapy department was on holiday leaving just a skeleton staff for emergencies. So apart from my own efforts at keeping my muscles working, I had very little exercise for those few days. Just how much I was going to suffer for this, I had no idea, but believe me, I was soon to find out!

The day came when my ambulance arrived at the door and took me once more on my circular route to the hospital, to start once again my visitations to the girls in brown. I made my way gingerly on my crutches and waited my turn for treatment. As I sat there I thought of my earlier efforts at exercising, and wrongly lulled myself into thinking that I was going to have a similar experience. Well as it turned out, I was sitting there in a dream world all of my own making.

'Mr Hill? Raymond Hill?' a voice gently brought me back to reality.

'Yes dear,' I said, as I struggled to my feet with the aid of my crutches. I took a few stumbling steps and entered the 'torture chamber'. The sweet young thing that had called me in now helped me out of my trousers and into a pair of shorts. So here I was, all ready for action. I lay back on the top of the plinth, and between us we took off the bandages and removed the splint. We both looked at what was now a decidedly nasty sight.

The knee itself was badly swollen and looked a multi-coloured mess. I had half expected this from the pain I had felt for the past few days, but the sight of my quadriceps was something that I had not thought to see. For you just couldn't see what wasn't there, and that was the reason for my dismay. I had no muscles, just flab. It was obvious that there was no strength in them. My dismay must have shown clearly in my expression, for my physio felt gently around the leg and then, in a kindly voice, said, 'Don't worry Mr Hill, we have a long way to go but if we both help each other, we will most certainly win.' Here was another confident young lady ready for action.

Time could not be wasted so we threw ourselves into action. The first thing we had to do was just quad exercises, but first of all we had find the damn things. For the first few visits there seemed to be no response at all to our joint efforts, but then, ever so slowly, my muscles came back to life, and enough to let me start leg raising. From then onwards, there seemed to be nothing but progress, I could tighten my muscles and do straight lifts virtually at will.

So came the time for me to see the surgeon so that he could check on my progress so far. I saw him in the outpatients' clinic, and that in itself was an experience. You could take a packed lunch and stay there all day. I was lucky, my name was soon to be called, and in I went, crutches and all. He wasn't over the moon at the state of the knee, but he sanctioned the commencement of knee bending.

I turned up at my next physiotherapy appointment already knowing the worst. We weren't going to like it from now on, especially me!

'Are we ready then,' my little brownie said. As it turned out she was ready, I was ready, but the bloody knee certainly wasn't! It seemed to be set as if in concrete, with granite chippings mixed in as well for good measure. All early efforts achieved nothing except cries of pain and anguish, all from me, not the physiotherapist. Oh how I hated that knee.

Gradually, after many visits, we forced the thing to bend very slowly, but at least it was progress of a sort. We pressed ahead with the full series of knee bending and quads exercises. I was always glad at the end of every session to get back to the comfort and safety of my splint and bandages. After numerous visits I was able to be rid of my crutches and graduate to walking sticks. Week after week went by and with visits three times a week I was making progress, but not enough for me to go into the large quads class with the other lads. Each week saw me gain more and more strength, with more muscle and knee bending, until eventually, after five months from the date of my operation, I was discharged.

Here I was, home once more, out of hospital again, and we all wondered whether this was the last time.

14

I had eighteen months, then the all too familiar pains in my groin started up again, and took me off to the doctor. It was a quick trousers down!

'Cough. Hernia. Hospital!'

It turned out to be a very short stay, and at least it was a different hospital. Even the operation was a mere formality and of little consequence. Then ten days in hospital, four weeks rest, then back to work. Easy!

15

It was about two years later, this was 1968, that I started to feel ominous danger signs in my knees again, yes both of them. At first, minor aches and pains, which in no time at all developed into constant pain at all times. Kneeling was hell, and using the clutch in the car with the left leg was even worse! My knees were terribly painful, and this gradually got worse as the weeks passed by, until, in the end, I had to capitulate and go and see my doctor. He promptly despatched me to the hospital yet again. It was the same hospital where I had my kneecaps scraped, so at least I would be in surroundings that I knew.

My first surprise was that I had a new consultant, as my last one had moved on to another hospital in the area. Ah well, I told myself, it will be a different opinion, so that should be a good thing. As usual, I sat in the main hall waiting to hear my name being called out. That time duly arrived, and in I went. I was shown to my cubicle and told to strip off and wait for the consultant to arrive with his crew. This time it was going to be different, as I soon found out. A nurse arrived with a multi-coloured robe and said, 'Just slip this and your shoes on, and follow me.' As I slithered along behind her, I thought what a bony specimen I must have looked, I hoped I wouldn't meet anyone I knew. Wasn't I in for a shock.

'Here we are, Mr Hill,' said the nurse as she tapped on the door. I followed her in. I was absolutely shattered, for the surgeon was there all right, but so were at least thirty student doctors and physiotherapists.

'Kindly slip off your robe and shoes, and lie on the plinth,' he told me in a quiet but confident voice. I felt better already, even though, to tell the truth, I felt a right twit with everyone staring at me.

'Now then Mr Hill, what seems to be the problem? Take your time and in your own words.' With this, he started to examine both my legs from top to bottom.

I would have liked to have shouted out loud that it was my bloody kneecaps giving me constant pain, but why should I, it wasn't his fault that I had played too much sport and had stopped too many hard cricket balls with my legs rather that a bat! So instead I said, 'It is severe pain behind the kneecaps, and any knee movement increases the pain.' He nodded in agreement as he bent both my legs and felt my muscle reaction, or lack of it. I also explained my crouching problem; I could hardly bend my knees at all, no more slip fielding, that was for sure. Now he was gently rotating my kneecaps, and even though he was not applying much pressure, I was in agony and it obviously showed in my ashen features.

'Bloody Nora!' I murmured quietly to myself, only not quiet enough, hence quite a few sniggers from the audience.

'Sorry Mr Hill, both your patellas will have to come off.' He called some students forward to examine my knees. I couldn't have had a bigger shock if he had said some other 'twosome' of my anatomy were to be removed.

'What do you mean, come off?' I asked in a rather shocked and incredulous voice.

'Well it is a similar operation to the ones you had when you had your scrapes, but much more final.' I lay there in a state of shock for a few moments, then asked in a quiet voice, trying to be as calm as possible.

'When will you do it?'

'Well as soon as possible, for your patellas are of no use to you now, so I think the sooner the better.' He had a quietly comforting voice, 'Would you object to going to Oswestry for the operation?'

OSWESTRY! Where the hell is Oswestry, I thought to

myself, but I answered, 'No I don't mind, I will go anywhere.'

'Good, we will be able to fit you in very quickly. We will let you know how soon by letter.' With that information I left him and all his students to discuss me and my kneecaps.

It was only when I got home and looked in my AA car book, that the problem of going to Oswestry dawned on me. It was at least seventy miles from my home, what had I let my family in for? I hoped it wouldn't be for too long. My wife and I both agreed that it would be worth it, just to remove the painful kneecaps would be worth the inconvenience caused.

I kept going to physiotherapy for exercises until February 1969, when I was called, and I was on my way to yet another hospital. It was bitterly cold, with snow and icy conditions everywhere. Now, to get to Oswestry to be admitted was almost like going to the North Pole. I started off with a fifteen mile bus journey, from Poynton to Manchester, and from there I boarded a coach at 10 a.m. This coach was the only way for visitors, who didn't have their own transport, to get to the hospital to visit the patients there.

As we stood about on that cold morning, it was a wonder we didn't all get frostbite! If we thought that was bad, we were all in for a rude awakening. The coach eventually arrived, and I took one look at it and I knew, bad legs or not, I should have started to walk the seventy miles. At least the movement would have kept my circulation flowing. But no, like sheep we all piled into the vehicle and off we went. It didn't take many miles for us all to realise that the bloody contraption had no heater, or I should say it did have one but not in working order. So it was a case of pull your coat tightly about you, get your nose into a book or paper, and be brave and hope that time would pass quickly by. My thought was that when we were out in the country and away from the thirty mph zones, the driver would put his foot down and the miles would fly by, weather permitting. Pass thirty miles an hour? We couldn't even reach it, let alone pass it.

114

The miles dragged wearily on, with first one stop and then another. It was one continuous engine failure after another, due to the freezing conditions. It was so cold that your breath froze on the windows. Eventually, after taking four hours for a 70-mile journey, we arrived at the hospital. At least with me being a patient I didn't have to worry about the return trip later in the day. Thank God I didn't bring my family with me.

So this was Oswestry. I stood at the entrance and looked around at the rows of single storey buildings and the snow covered gardens and trees, and thought that even in the winter and frozen solid, it looked a very pleasant place indeed, as hospitals went, that was.

I picked up my bag and limped my way in. The signs told me as I moved along, that the large building on my left was the nurses' home, and on my right there was a small private patients' unit. Just past this I turned right, and stood at the entrance to an extremely long corridor. It looked endless and at first glance, seemed to stretch for miles. As I made my way along it with the other people off the coach, some visitors, and some like myself, new admissions, I noticed some ward names – Crewe, Denbigh etc – all pointing to the fact that this was the Welsh border area. Then success, there was the sign, 'Admissions'. I presented myself, 'Ray Hill from the MRI.' A quick look at the entry list.

'Ah yes, you are going into Goodford ward,' he said. Now I knew that I hadn't noticed that name on my walk so far.

'Which is that?' I asked the porter.

'Back to the main corridor and then turn right, then it's the last ward on your right. Go there and ask for Sister Jones,' he told me. Now there's a strange Welsh name, I thought, I'll bet there are more Welsh Jones's than there are Welsh hills, especially in this hospital.

Up with my bag again and off in search of pastures new. His directions were perfect, and in a few short minutes I reached my destination. So far so good, the only interruption to the walk was that on passing the door marked 'Physiotherapy' on my left, I was nearly flattened by three

115

girls in white uniform. How strange I thought, that they are not wearing brown like at the MRI. I half smiled to myself as I remembered some of my past experiences associated with that name. I wonder if I would have smiled had I known what lay ahead of me.

I entered my new ward by way of a short corridor. Just off this was a kitchen, the smell from which reminded me that I was still very cold and hungry, and the Sister's office, then it led into the large ward proper. I was immediately highly impressed, it was nearly all glass and shining bright. It was indeed the most pleasant hospital surroundings that I had so far encountered.

A pleasant voice in my ear said, 'Can I help you please Mr . . .?' I turned to see a very smart and attractive young woman in a lavender coloured uniform. 'I am Sister Jones, you must be Mr Hill.'

'Yes, that's me Sister,' putting down my bag and blowing on my hands, for as yet I hadn't warmed up from my freezing trip.

'Have you been brought in your own transport, or on the Manchester bus?' she asked.

'The bus, if you can call it that.' I then explained about the ill-fated journey and my semi-freezing state.

'We will fix you up with hot food and drink, and then I will take down your particulars.' Now that didn't sound like a bad start to me, whichever way she meant it!

As good as her word, I was soon warm and full, having eaten an excellent meal in the ward kitchen. Things were getting better every minute. The Sister then took me to the top of the ward and showed me my bed. She told me to stay dressed until the visitors had left. It was a lovely ward with clear views of the gardens, and even though they were now covered with snow, you could imagine them in the summer with the lovely borders and roses. Still, I wouldn't see any of that, for I would be long gone before the spring even. If only I knew what lay ahead of me!

The bell to end visiting time at last was rung, and after everyone had gone, I turned to introduce myself to my new companions. I was pleased to find that both young and old were all very friendly and cheerful, despite their different ailments. Again, there was the feeling of guilt as I looked around at the bodies that were encased in plaster, legs strung on high, artificial joints etc., and here was me, with nothing but a slight limp to tell them that anything was wrong with me. The following months were going to remove that feeling of remorse for ever, but I wasn't to know that yet, not by a long way.

I made my round of the ward, the toilets, the bathroom and sluice. I just couldn't believe it. Comparing S1 at the Manchester Royal Infirmary to Goodford was just impossible to imagine. It was like comparing a Morris Minor to a Rolls Royce.

Everything that followed was the usual hospital routine, supper, drug round, late night drink, and then sleep until your early morning call of, 'Good morning gentlemen, wakey wakey.' This was the cry of the night nurses. Now I was an early riser, so when I was able I used to help out with the drink trolley, and the washing up which followed. First, it helped out, and secondly, it helped to get to know everyone in the ward. My only unwritten law was: no please or thank you, no drink. It worked wonders for bad manners.

In Goodford the early morning banter between both patients and patients, and patients and nurses, told me I was in a happy ward. The lads were from near and far, London, Shrewsbury, Birmingham, Manchester, and all parts of Wales, but fortunately we had one thing in common – laughter. Oh yes, lots of pain and agony to be suffered, but nearly always there was laughter echoing around the ward. My nearest companion was an old Irishman who was in for a hip replacement operation, but before he could have it, he had to stop smoking, and as he smoked sixty a day, it was not going to be easy. Every time he coughed, he had a fall of soot. There was also a lad from Manchester who had severe muscular problems, but he had a heart as big as a cabbage and unlimited courage. There was a Daily Express sports writer from Birmingham with a very badly

117

broken leg, but with a smile a mile wide and a locker full of booze. He certainly had no trouble with his water works! My fourth close companion was a Lancashire lad who was well on the way to recovery after a bad spinal operation that had certainly not affected his sense of humour. It was one continuous 'have you heard this one?' from one side of the ward to the other, followed by howls of laughter, with the staff failing to control us, especially if Sister was missing.

The procedure at this hospital was that you were operated on by your own consultant from Manchester, or wherever you had come from, then the Oswestry staff took over your welfare. It seemed to work perfectly. I was lucky, my surgeon was said to be very capable, very quiet, but first class. He came along with his entourage to see me and plan his campaign. They surrounded my bed, and they all had a long chat about my troublesome knees, everyone seemed to want to examine them. The consultant took me by complete surprise when he asked, 'Which one would you like me to take first?' First! I was dumfounded, so in complete ignorance I asked if both could be done at the same time. This simple remark was greeted with grins all round, and the surgeon telling me that there was no chance of that at all. It would have to be one at a time. Well in the end I opted for the right one, for no apparent reason because both were as bad as each other, but we had to start somewhere. I wasn't to be long waiting for a completely new experience in my hospital life (my sixth so far).

The time passed quickly by, for I busied myself in all manner of ways to keep my mind off tomorrow, and what was to come – letter home, cards, jokes and dominoes. Tea came and went, but I had no appetite for I was now very apprehensive about my operation. To seem outwardly calm, I lay there on my bed reading and smoking a cigar. I was disturbed by the arrival of two nurses armed with a trolley containing plastic gloves, a jug and a bucket. What now, I wondered. Bed bath? Enema? No, none of these things, it was my bed that was going to be washed down, I couldn't believe it. I was sent off for a quick bath myself, which I had, and returned to see my bed completely stripped down, and they were washing everywhere, including the wheels. When they had finished and remade the bed, it was spotless and much too nice to lie on, so I sat down in a chair, but not for long. The nurses pulled the curtains round the bed and uttered the command, 'Now in there and take your pyjamas off this instant!'

'With both of you?' I cried in an incredible voice, so all and sundry could hear, though I did as I was told. I was given a back to front operation gown, and a fig leaf.

'What gives girls? My operation isn't until the morning.' They then explained how the pre-operation system worked at Oswestry. It seemed that I would be taken from Goodford, all the way back up the corridor to the operating ward, where I was going to spend the night before the deed was done, and then I was to remain there for 24 hours afterwards. I thought how strange this was, a feeling I still have to this day.

Everything had been done and I was ready for the off.

'Everything ready nurse?' It was the voice of Sister Jones who had appeared with my notes and x-rays, a folder that was getting quite heavy as the years passed.

'Can I have your rings and watch and I will keep them for you. Now what about your teeth?' She looked serious but I wasn't sure.

'I may be going bald and have to wear glasses all the time, but my teeth are good and they are my own, so you can't bloody well have them at all.'

'Off you go, out of my ward.' She waved me off disdainfully.

'Wait a minute,' and I made a grab for my cigars.

'Oh no, just this,' and she handed me my toilet bag.

I shouted, 'Cheerio lads, see you when I see you.'

A voice shouted back, 'Every one in four doesn't come back,' followed by a sad cry of, 'goodbye number four.'

The two nurses wheeled me out of the ward and into the corridor, and we made our way towards the distant end. Unfortunately, some hospital beds are like supermarket

119

trolleys and have minds of their own, and this one was no exception. We made it, only through the hard work of my escorts, as we bounced from wall to wall. Little did I know it, but the sooner they got me to my destination, the sooner they were off duty. We went through the doors very quietly!

I immediately heard it, the sounds of moaning and people heaving as they tried to be sick. The girls, on direction from a Sister, pushed my bed into a space on the left-hand side of the ward, and there, directly opposite me, were all the beds of patients who had been operated on that day. Some silent and still, others in all kinds of trouble, but being nursed by several Sisters. It almost seemed as if there was a Sister to each bed, so good was all the attention being paid to their needs. My two nurses left me with whispered good luck messages.

'Hello Mr Hill, you aren't too worried are you?' She sounded reassuring.

'Not really Sister, but I must admit it is really off-putting.' I waved my arm to the other side of the ward. She explained that the hospital could look after the surgical cases before and after the operation, more completely and carefully if they were all in the same ward, under the close attention of highly skilled and experienced nursing Sisters. Everyone was together in this ward, male and female adults, and also the children. I didn't like the idea then, or later.

I lay there staring at the ceiling, trying not to listen to all the noise. Roll on sleep, I thought. Well help came in that way with the arrival of yet another Sister Jones, with a glass of milk and two sleeping tablets.

'Thanks Sister,' and I immediately got my head down.

It seemed only minutes later that I was gently being shaken awake by a smiling orderly. A whispered good morning, and have a quick wash for me. I looked about, and said a quiet good morning to the lads on either side of me. Both, it seemed, were cartilage operations, so all three of us were leg jobs, and all three of us were MRI patients. The clock on the wall hadn't yet reached six o'clock, and there we were, all washed and waiting. I was trying not to think too much about food and drink, for I was starving. Bragging, I said I could eat a man and his horse, and then it seemed that they were more frightened than I was. Apparently, this was the first time in hospital for both of them so I tried to console them.

'Don't worry lads, this is my third leg operation.' If they had only known that for two pins I would have jumped out of bed and made a run for it!

'Mr Hill?' I turned, and there stood looking over me was a tall slim nurse in blue, and wearing a mask and glasses. 'Time to prepare your leg for the theatre.' She surrounded me with screens, and then brought her trolley in with her.

'Down flat,' she ordered as she rolled down the bedcovers. She then started to carefully place towels under the leg and went ahead and carefully shaved it. That was from the very edge of my fig leaf to my toes. She had made a perfect job of it, and there was no trace of blood whatsoever.

'Well done miss,' I started to say, but a brusque retort shut me up very quickly.

'Nurse, if you don't mind.'

'Sorry, nurse.' That put me in my place all right.

'Now this is the part I really like best,' she said from behind her mask, where I think she was smiling. Splosh! She hit my thigh with a large swab, expertly held with forceps. It was freezing! In a flash, with quick smooth strokes and continuous replenishing of the yellow antiseptic solution, there I was, with a definite Far Eastern colouring to my leg, feet and toes. She held her swab in the air, and gave her handiwork an appraising look.

'Oh dear, missed some,' and she quickly made a long firm stroke up the inside of my leg. My hands hastily covered my fig leaf, I didn't mind one ice-cold yellow leg, but that is as far as it goes.

'Chicken,' was all she said, and then very thoroughly covered my leg in a criss-cross pattern, with sterilised sheets.

'That is you completed,' she said, and removed her mask. She was a very attractive girl with, as I thought, a very nice smile.

'Are you from Manchester, or a local girl?' I asked.

'Oldham, and before you ask, yes I do know.' And off she swept with her trolley. Cheeky monkey.

'Good morning, and thanks very much nurse.' I gave her a cheery wave and settled back to see what the rest of the day had to offer.

My eyes took in the other side of the ward, and yesterday's victims. I counted the beds, they were all still full, that was comforting, more to them than me. Now I was green with envy, as those who wanted it had tea and toast. Mind you, there weren't many takers, but oh, what I would have given for the tea. It was strange to hear the voices of women and children crying out for nurses, in what seemed to be, from our end at least, an all male ward. Then above the general noise of the ward, I heard conversation and peals of laughter coming through a doorway across the room. It was the same doorway from which I received a visitor. It was the anaesthetist.

'Good morning.' He seemed a nice guy. He gave me a quick examination. 'First class,' he told me. I hope we can say that in the morning, I thought to myself. It was only a short time later that I had another visit. This time a Sister with my pre-med. injection. She was very competent and I felt only a slight prick.

'Now lie back and relax, for you are the first on the list this morning.' I was certainly glad of that anyway, and soon I was feeling drowsy and very dry mouthed. I didn't fight it for I had learnt that it is very much better just to drift along with it. I was disturbed only to be helped onto the theatre trolley.

'Can you slide over for us Raymond, there's a good lad.' I helped as best I could, and was soon on my way. As I looked up into the porter's face, I just managed a sly wink.

First stop was the anteroom for my knockout drop. I was feeling quietly very calm and ready for the injection in my hand. Then ten, nine, eight, then blackness. That feeling wasn't going to last, for the next thing I remember, I was yet again in a face slapping contest. Everyone seemed to enjoy this part, especially with me. Or so it seemed, and even in my half-dazed condition, I knew what was required, so I spat out the 'mouth organ'. For then the slapping stopped. I was a quick learner!

'Well done Raymond.' Then I was sick again. Oh boy, was I sick. I heaved and heaved! Even before a distant voice told me to, I was taking in great gulps of air, but as usual, that didn't help me either. I felt bloody dreadful, I was weak and sweating pints, and worse than that, I was still being sick. No matter how many operations I had, I found that I could handle the pain, but the sickness was sometimes too much.

In my muddled thoughts, I thought I heard a voice calling, 'Mr Hill, can you hear me?' This question seemed to be repeated over and over again. I opened my eyes, and there at the end of the bed, was a figure in white. My muddled brain put the pain and sickness together and I thought that it might well be an angel who had come for me. I tried to focus my watery eyes on this vision, and then it dawned on me, it was only a damned physiotherapist. Stupid bitch, what does she want? Then it all clicked; I knew what she wanted, and I knew what I wanted, but I knew she would not go away until she had won. She didn't have to ask or tell what she required me to do, so with a very great effort, I forced the bandaged leg up off the bed until my toes touched the top of the cage which held the sheets up off my leg.

'Well done Mr Hill, well done!'

From me she got a rude, 'Sod off', which unfortunately for me, was heard by the Sister.

'I will put that outburst down to pain and frustration.' Even while she was talking to me, I was reaching for the bowl, heaving and heaving. Then my chastiser became my caring Sister.

Always, every second that passed, there seemed to be someone there to mop your brow and care for you. I had no idea how long it had been since my operation, but the pain was beginning to come through. I gritted my teeth and tried to stick it out, but it was no use.

'Sister, please help me?' She told me that I would soon be given an injection that would make me sleep and, as good as her word, my injection came and I was soon in a deep and heavy slumber.

How long I had been out I had no idea, but as I opened my eyes and peered about me, I was pleased to find that in spite of the pain, the sickness had gone, at least for the time being. Just as quickly though, I knew that my leg was much worse, but I supposed that was only to be expected. At least now I felt that I wanted to take a clearer look around me, so I felt on top of my locker for my glasses. Putting them on, I glanced sideways at the two lads next to me, who were having their operations later. Both were sleeping soundly. Good for them, they seemed to be having no trouble at all. Looking at the clock, I found that it had turned one o'clock – lunchtime. The mere thought of it made me start heaving again. Was there no bloody end to this.

I did think, though, that I could murder a cup of tea. No sooner the thought, than a charming orderly came across the ward.

'I have just been feeding the others,' she said, as she waved her hand across the other side of the room. 'Can I get you anything, a slice of toast, tea, coffee or juice?'

'I will settle for a cup of tea please, that can't do me any harm.' I must have been joking! She brought the tea in a beaker, and I drank it very carefully. Within seconds I was in trouble again. I just heaved and heaved, and was violently sick again. Still, it took my mind off my leg, because that was now bloody murder, and was getting worse all the time. I kept a wary eye on the door and thought that if a physiotherapist made a move towards me, I would clobber her with my empty urine bottle.

As I lay staring at the ceiling and trying to put the pain out of my mind, and at the same time, taking big deep breaths to try vainly to control the sickness. I thought, bloody Nora, three surgical knee operations, and one to go.

I will be glad when that one is done, and then it will be all over. Hells bells, if only I knew what lay before me. Again.

Soon there was a distraction that helped me to pass the time away, the exodus of the previous day's victims. Beds were wheeled out in convoy, all going to their individual wards. All that seemed to be missing was John Wayne at the head, shouting, 'Wagons roll!'

As is always the case, the time ticked away, and in between sleeps and various injections, the night passed away quite uneventfully. Even so, as soon as I awoke, I knew that I still couldn't face food or drink, so I left well alone. All the action in the ward was on the other side, where today's victims were all being prepped by the nurse. She seemed so calm and efficient, but I still wondered whether this was the best way to do it, spending so long in a ward like this. To hospital beginners, I think it could be a bit overpowering. Wasn't taking you from your own ward and surroundings, to the theatre, and then straight back to the same place, a much better idea? It certainly seemed to be the better way to me.

At last, time to go! Two nurses had arrived to take me on my long journey back to Goodford. On the way back, I noticed once again that there were many more girls in white than in nurse's uniform. I was yet to realise why. My nurses whisked me back to the ward in no time at all.

16

There were cries of 'Welcome home!' and also other remarks as well from my friends, for all were names long since forgotten, but faces never. All the people, patients, nurses, physios and doctors are still remembered years later.

Sister paid me a visit, and with the help of one of the nurses, made me comfortable, a clean pyjama top, talcum powder, and a wash and shave. I felt better already. A jug of water was placed on my locker, and an empty urine bottle by the bed.

'Empty that, and fill that, or else!' Sister said. It was only then that I realised that I hadn't passed water since my operation.

'Oh hell, not again,' I moaned, 'I will drink some now please.' And very dutifully I downed a full glass of water. I had sensed that I was going to have trouble with my leg, so I was very determined that nothing else would go wrong.

A little while passed in friendly banter with my comrades, again the feeling of finding out that hospital is a great leveller. For it mattered not who you were, how high or how low outside, once you were in your pyjamas, you were a patient. My ward philosophy was soon disturbed by visitors, two of them, one a physiotherapist, and the other the registrar, a Cape Coloured South African – a man over the next few months I was going to learn to admire and respect, and also to have plenty of laughter with. He was an icon.

'How are you Mr Hill?' he asked.

'Not too bad at the moment, but that will change when she starts on me,' I replied, and smiled at his companion.

'Don't worry, all I am going to do for the time being is to keep this one in good condition, ready for when you are walking about.' With this, she placed her hands on the quads of my left leg, her hands were freezing.

'Well will you warm your hands before you start please,' I said then added 'Also be careful where you put those cold hands!' The poor lass actually blushed. They covered me up again and left.

Twenty-four hours went by, the sickness had gone, but the pain in the knee was something else! There was good news though, I had been able to fill my bottle, what an achievement! Everyone was delighted. I had also managed to eat some breakfast, and much more important, keep it down. Things were going great, almost too good to believe.

Ward rounds took place, and various surgeons and doctors checked on their own patients. In my case, my South African friend arrived accompanied by my Sister. He looked at the large mound of bandages, then placed his brown hands on my thigh, and asked me to tighten my quads. I did my best. 'How about a lift?' he asked.

'Why, where are we going?' I couldn't resist it.

'Funny man,' he smiled, but then he got his own back. 'Now lift!'

I lay back and grabbed the bedsides, and tried like hell. I struggled hard, but failed dismally. All I had done was to disturb that 'sleeping giant' – pain. It was like dropping a heavy stone in a pool and feeling the ripples of sheer agony spread out from the knee to all parts of my leg.

'Steady now, that will do. Don't go mad,' Sister said, and off they went. Well, I thought to myself when they had gone, there is nothing really to worry about because they can't do anything to me that I haven't had before, and I came through that all right. My God, how wrong I was.

Oswestry was different to anywhere for their physiotherapy. There seemed to be as many physiotherapists as there were nurses, if not more. They were like bees, they swarmed all over the wards. They always seemed to appear after breakfast when everything was cleared away. There

127

were tall ones, short ones, thin ones and fat ones, and some real beauties, but all were exceedingly pleasant, and all worked like beavers.

It appeared that I was to share my young lady with the guy in the next bed. He had had a back operation, but was due to go home in a couple of days. From behind the curtains I could hear all the moans and groans as she went to work on his muscles, for possibly the last time. Also coming from behind there was the sound of laughter, male and female. There it was again, laughter, the magic medicine.

Now it was my turn. 'Good morning Raymond,' she smiled, as if in anticipation of the things she had in store for me.

Here we go again, I thought to myself, but out loud I said,

'Good morning dear.' I needn't have worried, for the time being it was a cakewalk. Gentle raising of the right leg, and much more energetic work on the left.

'We need to work hard on this left leg and get it in good condition for all the extra work that lies ahead of it.' Neither or us realised as she made the remark, that it was to be the understatement of the year. I was soon to learn the physiotherapist's war cry 'No pain, no gain,' the hard way. And to find out that it only takes one small step to change the therapist to terrorist.

The next few days went by with just the normal simple exercises, but with an increasingly nagging thought in my mind. The pain in the right knee was getting worse all the time, or so I thought, but I decided to keep quiet about it, for it was nearly stitch removal time. Just one more day to go.

The following day, Sister duly arrived with her trolley. She soon had the bandages and splint removed to reveal yet another swollen and badly discoloured knee for all to see. It was obvious this time that it was filled with fluid, and not a pretty sight. But, thank God, it was nowhere near as bad as my experience in the MRI.

'Trust you to be awkward,' she declared, as she gently covered the trouble area. She then departed. On her return she was accompanied by the registrar, who had a good look and decided that the stitches could still be taken out. Nineteen in all, with never the removal of one felt. A magic job, all things considered.

'If Sister and your physiotherapist don't get that swelling down I will have to aspirate it,' he said. 'I will give them a couple of days.' My raised eyebrows, with the talk of them removing the swelling, went unnoticed or ignored!

Unfortunately, all efforts failed, so therefore the time came for the needle to go in and the fluid to be removed. I was not looking forward to this one little bit, for it was only twelve days since the operation, and the knee was still bloody painful! But I needn't have worried at all, for I hardly felt a thing, considering the state it was in.

All that was the easy part, and that ended there and then! The joint was locked solid. There was no bend at all, and my quadriceps were in a terrible state. So, for both my physiotherapist and myself there started numerous hours of hard work, both in the ward and in the department (the torture chamber.) It was a double-barrelled attack, for on my right leg it was ice packs and all things to do with getting the swelling down and the bruising away, and also gentle quads exercises. But on the left leg it was a very, very different story, for the physiotherapist launched herself at it with weights, springs and continuous P & F (Proprioceptive Neuromuscular Facilitation) exercises. It was hammered mercilessly to give it the supporting strength it was going to need. It was work, work and more work. This went on day after day after day. At the end of each session I was completely and utterly knackered. The girls would bring me back from the department, and throw me on my bed, a complete wreck.

17

It was about this time, as I and others like me were struggling and fighting with the dedicated physiotherapists, that I saw the downfall of the other type of patient, the 'malingerer'. This one was from the MRI also. He supposedly had a bad back and couldn't work, and hadn't for three years. All of us thought it was a funny ailment, for on ward rounds or with physios, he couldn't manage a move without cries of agony. Yet on other occasions when there were no staff about, he could stretch from out of his bed, down into his locker for cigarettes or beer, or even walk about with no apparent difficulty. He may have been able to kid a lot of people, but here in Oswestry he was not going to kid anyone, especially our MRI surgeon who was of different stock than medical people he had dealt with before.

He had been in Goodford a week when a full ward round was on. There was the surgeon, registrar, Sister and physiotherapist. The consultant, a small and seemingly mild man, stood at the end of his bed. We were all able to see and hear what followed. Quietly, he asked the patient, 'How is your back today Mr . . .'

His answer, a moaned, 'I can't move it doctor,' was answered very sharply and loudly.

'Get up now, get dressed and leave this hospital this minute, and make your own way back to Manchester. All our x-rays, tests and physiotherapy reports show you to be a fraud and a malingerer.' He added, 'There is absolutely nothing wrong with your back that exercise, and most of all, some work, won't put right.' And then to Sister, 'By the end of this ward round I want him out of here.' It was an instruction she was happy to comply with. Well done Doc.

For the rest of us there was pain and then more pain. But also there was so much fun, laughter was always ringing around the ward, more often than not at a poor nurse's expense. Anything they said in innocence was quickly turned around to mean something different, and more often very rude!

On one occasion Sister decided that she would straighten my bed after I had been seen and examined by the registrar. She reached right under my cage to reach my sheets, but instead all she reached was my 'private' parts!

'Sister,' I shouted in mock horror, 'what are you doing?' Her blushing departure from the ward at full speed was hilarious.

On Goodford ward we were blessed with a nursing nun, she was always dressed in white, and everyone respected her. There were never rude jokes in her earshot, she was a truly wonderful person.

Now, by this time I was making my own way, on crutches, to and from the department which was only a little way from the ward. Now a crutch, carefully aimed, can be a deadly weapon to any nurse or physiotherapist behind curtains drawn around a bed, though only when he knew the medical condition of the patient, or what else was going on. 'Bum rub' was always the best time. 'Bum rub', these two words cover a whole multitude of different approaches to this part of the nurse's tender loving care, an important side of their profession, especially in an orthopaedic hospital. Broken and sore skin on a patient's pressure points can cause absolute agony on long-term bed patients. Nurses have their own different ways to this carry out this task. First, there is the hard case, the man-hater. She is the one who would be happier rubbing a man's pressure points with a sanding block. Also, she is the one whose attitude would be completely the opposite if she were rubbing female pressure points. Then there are the girls who are most efficient and caring, and do the job quickly with no shown

131

emotion, in the true sense of nursing. That leaves, lastly, the sultry temptress type of nurse, the one who knows she is a real seductress of the highest order. She can do more with her gentle caressing fingertips, to your 'bum' than an expert geisha girl from the Orient. All the time that this is going on, her innocent face bears no emotion, none whatsoever. Needless to say, our 'nursing nun' was the very efficient type of nurse. She was an angel in white.

Now, one morning I was hobbling back from treatment in the physiotherapy department, after yet another battering, when I saw that most of the beds were surrounded by curtains. I thought that here was a chance to liven things up a bit, so I swung my way up the ward until I got near my own bed, and then I aimed for the nearest pair of legs I saw. Now trust me to cock it up! There was a scream, a clattering of a tray, and before I could reach my own bed, out came a very red faced nun. And even worse, she was followed from the other side of the bed by Sister, who tore me to ribbons. Quickly, I apologised to them both, and made my way to my bed to hide behind a book until things cooled down. Now I am always told that God pays debts without money, and my payment for my tomfoolery came very quickly.

The following morning I had a visit from a doctor I had never seen before, he was with one of our staff nurses, a titian-haired beauty. He quickly examined my right knee thoroughly, and indeed very roughly. Enough to arouse the 'demon' pain again.

'Mr Hill, I wonder if you would mind having your knee x-rayed for me? It is a special type of x-ray, called an arthogram. It would be the left leg, and it would certainly help the hospital teaching school.' I wasn't keen on him, but I agreed.

The staff nurse had been shaking her head from side to side, and mouthing silently the word 'no', but I had already said yes, and the doctor was on his way out. The staff nurse was furious, and said angrily, 'Do you know what you have let yourself in for Raymond?'

'Bloody hell, staff, it's only an x-ray,' I replied, 'Isn't it?'

'You will see, you will see.' She went away, shaking her head.

By this time I had graduated from the real hard exercises, to working in the gym, and best of all, in the hospital swimming pool. This was one of the treats of a hospital stay in Oswestry, to swim in a pleasantly warm swimming pool, with a lovely physiotherapist by your side. At this stage, my 'water ballet' movements were restricted purely to walking in the water (not on it) and to knee bending, by hanging on to the rails around the side. Both of these things came very easily in the pool, compared with the same efforts out of it.

Suddenly, my solace was interrupted by a shout from the pool-side. It was the department head. 'Raymond, you are needed in x-ray.' So with the help of my physio, out I got. I towelled myself dry and changed swimming trunks for shorts and dressing gown, had my leg re-bandaged and made my way to x-ray, feeling quite pleased with my progress on the crutches for that distance.

I presented myself to the receptionist who quickly ushered me through into the department. Two people were there waiting for me, a nice radiologist, and the doctor who wanted the pictures. They soon had me on the table with the left leg bared and ready for action.

It didn't take long for the doctor to place the needle in my knee just behind the patella, and then to inject the dye into it. This was required to help the girl take her pictures. It was by no means a pleasant experience, but I had suffered worse in the past. The knee hurt like blazes, but I closed my eyes and clenched my teeth, and hoped I wasn't showing how I felt. Then suddenly it was all over, and for me only just in time, for waves of nausea were beginning to roll over me, and I was already at the deep breathing stage. Then, that was the pictures taken, and the needle removed, much to my relief. But when I opened my eyes there was no sign of a doctor, only a very quiet x-ray girl who helped me off the table and passed me my crutches, with a quiet, 'I'm

133

sorry if we hurt you.' I gave her half a smile and hobbled away on what were now *two* very painful legs. It seemed miles back to the ward and I felt dreadful. I must have looked as bad, for I bumped into the Sister on the way back into the ward.

'You look like death!' she exclaimed. 'Go and get on your bed at once and stay there.' It was a tone of voice that wasn't going to be argued with. I did as ordered and was soon accepting gratefully the two pain-killers she brought me. 'At least that experience should keep you quiet and out of trouble for a while.' I didn't think that she felt as stern as she sounded.

The following morning I was in the pool again, by now my favourite place, with the water such a lovely temperature, and with the steam gently rising from the surface it was lovely and relaxing. But it was a place that also made you realise how lucky you were, when you saw the other poor cases around you. My thoughts were soon disturbed by the cry of 'X-ray Raymond, they want you again.' As I climbed up the steps and out, I wondered what the hell they wanted me for now, perhaps they are going to show me the x-rays or something.

On my arrival at the x-ray department the 'or something' was painfully obvious. I was shown straight into the same room, where this time there were three people waiting for me, the doctor and two radiologists. The doctor said 'I am sorry about this, but we need some more x-rays.' I looked at them in utter disbelief! I should have told him there and then to get stuffed, but I didn't.

'OK but hurry up and let's get it over with quickly.' I remembered my nauseous feelings of yesterday, and I was more scared of being sick than anything else. They had me ready and on the bed in no time. One girl swabbed my knee and the other girl offered the doctor a needle. 'We don't need that,' he said, very roughly, 'he's a man isn't he?' And then, 'You don't need a local anaesthetic for this do you?'

He had put me in a position of not being able to scream

out 'Of course I want the bloody thing!' and I couldn't, not now. I shook my head.

'No I will be all right, but please get on with it.' I had made a mistake, a big one. I hadn't realised that the bloody big needle was going to go in the exact same place as yesterday's injection. He couldn't miss seeing that, it was the centre of a large black bruise on the inside of the knee. Well at least today they had asked me about the anaesthetic, yesterday no one had bothered to. The needle entered my knee, and it was as if someone had driven a six-inch nail into my leg. It hurt, and it hurt like blazes. How I did not cry or scream out loud I will never know, for it was agonising. My eyes were fixed on the needle. I watched them insert the dye, after which we had to wait a few minutes, and then they started filming. The x-ray machine went up and over the knee, which still had the needle in it, and took some pictures from all different angles. Then, as had happened previously, we finished the job in silence. The doctor took out the needle, and didn't even say thank you; he just left the room like yesterday. He was an ignorant, arrogant swine. The girls were very quiet and I could tell they were both embarrassed, so I said nothing. I just took my crutches and hobbled away.

After what seemed an eternity, I reached Goodford, and made my way wearily to my bed, and flopped exhausted upon it. I hadn't said a word all the way up the ward; I just lay there on the verge of tears. Unknown to me, one of the lads had made a dash to the office. He was soon back, accompanied by the staff nurse. She took one look at me. 'Raymond, what have they done?' she asked. I looked down at my leg to see that it had bled, and all the blood had dried down the leg, and my knee was swelling rapidly.

'I will get the trolley and clean you up, and then you can get straight into bed.' I wasn't going to argue with that, I was completely knackered.

She came back with the trolley, and accompanied by my registrar. He examined my knee, had a few words with the staff nurse, and off he went. She cleaned my leg very carefully, gave me a couple of pain-killers, tucked me into bed, and told me to stay there and get some sleep.

That was the last time I heard about arthograms (at least for a good while), but it was strongly rumoured that there had been a heated confrontation between the two doctors, my South African, and the Australian swine.

It took a few days for the left leg to settle down, but even so, it was still hard work as usual with the right one. It had been a bit of a set-back, but we were winning the battle, and so it turned out that after four weeks I was sent home and transferred to the MRI as an out-patient yet again.

18

Pain is something all of us have to bear at sometime or another, especially women. If us men had to have babies, I am sure there would not be as many around. But the need is to try and fight it, or at least try and cope with it. This is a personal thing for all of us, there was me with my battle with my knees, and lots of others like me, or even worse. At the same time there are the 'others'.

This one in question was a Welsh guy who had a cartilage operation, but his lack of effort and will power neither helped him, nor more importantly, the physiotherapists. Both in bed exercise and the gym, as soon as he was left on his own he would stop completely anything that he had been told to do. The others and I would be hammering away, then watch him lie back and do nothing. To say he got up my nose was an understatement! We would keep having a go at him, but it was no use. There was no 'Welsh dragon' in him. But you only reap, in physiotherapy, what you sow.

He was eventually discharged by a disgusted surgeon, with a knee with no bend in it at all, and there never would be. What a pillock.

19

After only four years, I was back to the girls in brown, for three visits a week. This lasted about six weeks before I was told to report back to Oswestry in two weeks time, because my right leg, and especially the knee, was strong enough to support me whilst they operated on my left. Once more into the breach, dear friends.

When I returned, it was to a new ward, Crewe. This was situated at the opposite end of the corridor from Goodford, which was now a ladies' ward. It was miles from the physiotherapy department, but almost opposite the pre-operative ward. The ward had a tremendous atmosphere (as indeed did the whole hospital); once again they were a superb staff, and a good crowd of patients. There were four of us from Manchester, and we had all arrived via the visitors' coach. The journey this time was first class, the start of summer and the lovely countryside. What a change from my previous visit.

The four of us entered the ward like the four musketeers and we all had different complaints. A hammer toe, a cartilage, a dislocated shoulder, and me and my knees. We hit it off straight away, more so when they gave us the first four beds on the left-hand side as you entered the ward, all next to each other. They were asking for trouble for we all laughed like school kids, but I was the big brother because I was the only one who had been in hospital before, the three of them were beginners. So, as they asked me question after question, I realised that I could paint it any colour I wanted.

The following morning, Monday 13 May, 1968 (there was

138

the dreaded number again, it was a good job it wasn't Friday or I would have been off home), I had a visit from the registrar.

'Where have you been? We expected you weeks ago.'

'I can only come when the MRI send me, I can't just come on my own,' it was no use him telling me off. 'But I have brought these three with me.'

'Oh no, not four of you all like him,' he said to the others, as he pointed at me. I told him not to worry, as they were all first-timers and that I would look after them.

'Heaven help them, and me,' he groaned.

Tuesday morning came around, and with it the ward round by the MRI surgeon and his followers. He had a few words with each of my companions, and then it was my turn.

'Hello Mr Hill, we meet once again. It will be the final operation for you in the morning, and then you will be pain free once again.' He paused as he was leaving my side, 'By the way, thank you for the arthograms.' I shuddered at the thought, but said nothing.

Night-time came, and the hospital routine of both bed, and patient bath time, and off into the pre-operative ward. We all went together in a small convoy, virtually just across the corridor. I had been very good so far, and had not attempted to scare the lads in any way, for I could tell from their quietness that day, that all three of them were very apprehensive about what was to happen to them. And to tell the truth, although it was my ninth operation, I felt the same way they did.

Everything went according to plan, so we all spent one night and one whole day in the care of the Sisters, and then it was back to our own ward in our sick and painful state. I wasn't interested in anybody else because, as usual, I spent most of the time heaving my heart up into a receiver held by one of the nurses. This lasted a couple of days, and then I began to take notice of what was going on around me. The good thing I found was that we were all back together in the same places, and we lined up with a cartilage, a hammer toe, me, then the bad shoulder, and we were all suffering in our own way, and all coping with the pain differently.

The cartilage lad must have been in agony, for he was moaning all the time. I thought, if he is like this now, how will he react when a physiotherapist gets hold of him. The hammer toe lad was very quiet but looked terrified, and resembled a frightened rabbit in his unusual surroundings. The only problem the broken shoulder lad had, was that now his arm was plastered in a bent position, and heavy. Every time he moved to his left slightly, he was always in danger of falling out of bed. Then there was me with my left leg, and a departed kneecap. I was feeling quite pleased that my sickness had left me, and I was used to the pain that I had. I thought that this time it would be two or three weeks at the most, before I was out and back to Manchester again. So I was going to try and have some fun, even if it was at the expense of my companions.

The first thing I had to do though, was talk Sister into a mirror for my 'monkey pole'. This time for some reason, my bed was propped up with my feet about eighteen inches above my head. Consequently I could only see sideways with no vision to the front, or any distance up the ward. But with the mirror fastened to the chain holding my handgrip, I was able to see the entire ward and the gardens behind me. It was like a submarine periscope, and it was a huge help for me to see everyone in the ward and feel a part of the goings on.

Like Goodford, it was a happy ward, with always the sound of laughter in the room, and I was certain that I was going to try to add to it as the days went by. In the ward we had road accident victims, both car and motorbikes, and a couple of construction workers who had found out that climbing down ladders was still the best way from the top of the building to the bottom, falling was quicker but much more painful.

By this time the pain in the leg was very bad, but I was determined not to show it to my companions, so I asked

140

them how they felt. The arm lad was fine, or so he said, but the other two lads were showing definite signs of distress, especially the cartilage lad. He said he was in intense pain and wanted some pain-killers, which Sister gave him. The lad next to me, with his hammer toe, didn't seem too bad pain-wise, but the whole experience of being in hospital obviously scared him a lot, and he was very quiet.

The first day after the operation passed by quickly, as did the night. I didn't sleep much, but I did have my usual quota of tea. In the morning I had to have help with washing and shaving, as I had a tendency to slide down to the top of the bed, with my head almost through the bars. I found that breakfast was also a big problem, but with help I managed to eat most of it. I couldn't wait until nine o'clock for the arrival of the physiotherapists, to see what effect it would have on my friends.

You could hear the sound of female voices from the short corridor, and then they were upon us like a swarm of bees. They walked along, comparing the names on our charts to the cards they had with them. They were indeed a friendly lot. One young lady read my name and said, 'Ah, Raymond, you are mine.'

My reply was, 'Sorry, I don't know it, but if you sing it I will try and join in!' She burst out laughing, and the ice was broken for all of us.

'In fact, you are all mine, all four of you.'

She had little to do with the toe or the shoulder, except to show them how to keep the muscles supple on the injured limbs. Next, she went to the cartilage. He asked for the curtains to be drawn while she treated him. From the agonised cries from behind them, you would think she was killing him. She wasn't there long, and then it was my turn. I asked her to leave the curtains open. She rolled the sheets down onto my cage, to reveal once again a mound of bandages on a well-protected leg, but she started on the right leg first.

'We must work this leg, seeing as it is not too long since you had surgery.' She went through all the exercises that I

141

knew and had been doing at home. 'Very good,' she said, 'that is quite good for now.' My eyes never left her as she moved round to my left side. What was to follow, I knew I was not going to like one bit. I was very pleased when all she wanted to do was to check on my quads. She placed one hand on my thigh, above the bandages, and asked me to tighten and relax. We did this about a dozen times, then came the moment I dreaded.

'Now Raymond, I want you to do just one lift for me, just so high.' She held her hand about a foot above my toes. 'It is not going to be easy propped up like that, but will you give it a try?' I knew that lots of eyes were on me, so I had to put on a bold front, I was scared but dared not show it. I grasped the edges of the bed, tightened my muscles as best I could, and strained away. Christ! Is there no end to this, I thought, but I struggled as hard as I could. The leg was hurting like hell, and I wanted to cry out, but I didn't dare. Then, at last it began to move, so I forced it up to her hand. 'Good,' she said, as I lowered the leg back down gently onto the bed. 'Looking at these cards I don't have to tell you to keep trying your exercises. Remember, five minutes in every hour.' She remade my bed and left the ward.

The 'cartilage' cried out, 'She made me do that, that can't be right to hurt you like that, can it?'

'Oh yes it can,' I replied, 'you wait until morning, and you must practice all the time what she has shown you now.' I knew I was wasting my breath, for if it hurt at all he wouldn't do it.

The 'hammer toe' said, 'Mine was easy, just tightening my muscles, that's all I have to do. I would die if I had to do what you two have to do.'

I fixed him with my pretend sad eyes and said, 'Well it doesn't really matter in your case, does it?' And I left it at that. He jumped at the bait.

'Why not?' he pleaded, 'why doesn't it matter about me?'

'Well that operation is a dodgy one, and it nearly always goes wrong, and when that happens, it's goodbye toes!' With that I turned away to hide my face.

142

My 'shoulder' partner in the next bed said

'You are a lousy sod, he will believe you, he is that sort of a bloke.' Then he laughed out loud, he was as bad as I was.

We were interrupted by the arrival of a group of nurses.

'Come on you lot, it's outside you're going, beds and all.' This was great news for me, for I was an avid sun-worshipper. So out we all went into the gardens. It was great. It was only the end of May, but it was a beautiful sunny day. Every day after the ward round, we were nearly all pushed out into the sun.

Morning again, and the return of the physiotherapists. Once again 'cartilage' died a thousand deaths, he was almost screaming, and the girl lost her temper.

'You are not trying, and I'll bet you are not doing your exercises. If you don't start helping yourself, you will have to come down to the gym.' She looked at me for support.

'Bloody hell, you will know all about it then, they will murder you down there.'

I am sure we frightened him between us, for she had no more trouble with him. As for me, things seemed to be progressing well with my left leg. I could bend it a little so soon, and my leg raising was quite good also. My only failing seemed to be with my quadriceps. No matter how hard I tried I could not get a flicker out of them. My right leg was given strenuous exercises without much difficulty, but my quadriceps were not developing as they should. And it wasn't through any lack of effort on the part of my physiotherapist or myself.

The days flew by and soon the registrar told me that I could have my stitches out in the morning. After that I could be wheeled to the gym for far more rigorous exercises on the left quads.

'They will soon build you up down there Raymond, but well done so far.'

As promised, the following morning my bandages and splint were taken off, and there was the knee for all to see.

143

It was again badly swollen, but nothing like it had been in the past. Sister was as pleased as I was.

'Well done, you have had enough trouble.'

Twenty stitches came out and I hardly felt a thing thanks to the loving care of the NHS.

I had been in hospital for twelve days and as I looked at my knee I thought that a few more days hard work and I would be on my way back home to my family. It felt really good. The hammer toe and cartilage lads had had their stitches out too, with no cries from the first. The second was almost weeping, and begging Sister not to hurt him. She told him not to be a baby and removed his five stitches. All his moans and groans had been for next to nothing. Still, we all handle pain with a great deal of difference.

Now sad things happen, and friends made get well enough to go home, and sadly for me my three friends all went home the next day, to go back to the MRI as out-patients. We had only been together for two short weeks, and in that time, as both day and night companions, you become very close indeed. It could work the other way but in our case it didn't. I was really sad to see them go.

By now I had developed a nice frontal suntan. I had a dark brown head, face and chest, plus one tanned leg. I looked, I was told by the nurses, like a chocolate which was half milk, half plain. I really loved being out in the gardens for the weather was glorious. It was now that something strange started to happen with my right knee. Sometimes when I was doing my leg exercises I would draw my leg up into the bend position and then I would have to push it back down with my hands. It just wouldn't go back down on its own. I didn't mention it to anyone at all, because I hadn't been out of bed yet, and that was my next milestone. It wasn't my secret for long, I had a very good physiotherapist and though I didn't complain, when she started to exercise the leg she knew something was amiss, as it was now Monday morning and she hadn't seen me since Friday when it hadn't been as bad. So I said it had only happened over the weekend which was mostly true. She pressed my

144

leg down straight on the bed, and where my patella had been there was now a depression. With the knee pressed firmly down it was quite obvious. Yet again, the knee was very painful, deep down I knew I was in trouble again.

My physiotherapist reported her findings to the doctors on the ward round, and it was quickly decided that there would have to be a further operation on the right knee to investigate the cause of the problem. This was to be carried out the following day, Tuesday!

At about this time there was a diversion on Crewe ward. On the previous day, the Sunday bus had arrived and with it a really big guy, well over six feet and about sixteen stone. That he was a gentle giant was soon obvious to all of us, and as he circulated, chatting to everybody, he seemed to be great company. But when he was told by the registrar and Sister that he would have to have an operation, his whole manner changed drastically. He raised his fist and smashed the top of his locker. Broken glass went everywhere. (Later we found that he had split the top of it, what power!) Tactfully and sensibly, they left him for a while to calm down. Half an hour later Sister and the staff nurse came to give him a sedative injection. As soon as they got near him and he saw the needle in the tray, he went berserk. Up went his arms, waving wildly about, Sister and the tray went one way and staff went violently the other! As soon as they gathered themselves together and left the ward he soon became calm again, but he never took his eyes away from the ward entrance. So when he saw Sister, the registrar, a male nurse and a porter, he leapt out of bed waiting for them. After a real struggle, and then only with the help of another male nurse and porter, were they able to force him back onto his bed so that Sister could give him what we found out later was a very heavy sedative to put him out. It did, but only for about ten minutes. Then he was up and stumbled out of the ward clad only in his pyjamas.

We were later told that he had made his way out through the rose gardens and onto the road where he was followed by a doctor and two male nurses who were joined by an

145

ambulance and two men. He apparently staggered for over a quarter of a mile before collapsing. The doctor gave him another sedative and all of them then went, by ambulance, back to the MRI. What an episode, and how sad. Who would want to be in the medical profession? Not me, that's for sure.

20

This new operation was certainly going to be a shock for my family when they came on Sunday, but at least it would be over by then, and I would have a few days to get over it.

So that night it was back to the pre-op ward again and even the Sister said, 'Not you again. Three times in four months, you must really like it here.' I had my leg shaved again, at this rate I was having more leg shaves than haircuts. The only thing that I was not happy about was the fact that I was the last one on the lists, so after being awakened at 6 a.m. for a wash and shave and nothing else, no food or drink, I then had to wait until late afternoon for my pre-med. Shortly after that I was taken through to the anaesthetist's room where I was again recognised. 'What, you again!' Then the last thing I remembered was the counting.

Here we go again, face slapping time, and cries of 'spit it out!'. Ah, the wonders of medical science. I woke as requested with my head in a bowl as usual. This time I was more sick than ever, all through the night and all the next day. I felt dreadful. I was given an injection to relieve the sickness but it didn't work at all so I had to spend a second night in there. Nothing seemed to be going right. At least I knew something had been done for I now had both legs swathed in bandages and weighing a ton each.

The registrar came to see me and tried to explain what they had found, and more to the point what they had done about it. It appeared that they opened up my leg and bent the knee two or three times and everything seemed to be OK. But at what was going to be the last attempt, it

147

happened for them, so they knew the problem, but much more importantly, they knew how to stop it. What was happening, the registrar told me, was on the last knee bend, the tendons had rolled off, and to the inside of the joint. On closer scrutiny they could see that the tendons were fraying like a rope being pulled over a jagged rock. A few more bends, he said, and the tendons would have snapped. They repaired the tendons and then sewed them into a muscle on the inside of my thigh. Then they took them across my knee at an angle and fastened them to a muscle beneath my knee on the right. It all sounded very complicated to me, so he did a simple sketch on one of my tissues. He also explained that the knee would only be about 80 per cent of its original strength. After his description I wasn't surprised.

Eventually it was decided that I could go back to Crewe ward. Sister had kept my bed vacant for me and there were three more new faces for me to get used to, but that was OK by me. Sister knew that I was on a downer and that I needed cheering up, so she had my bed pushed immediately into the sunshine and placed near her office window where she could keep her eye on me, and the roses. She also let me have my physiotherapy exercises out there, for she knew that I loved the sun. These weren't strenuous for it was now going to be a slow process on my quadriceps in both legs, although I must admit that it did help doing both legs together. It was a case of just the tightening up of my muscles and slight leg raising, but nothing too strenuous.

The days just crept along until it was time for the stitches to come out. I crossed my fingers as they took off the bandages and splints from both legs. The left knee was now looking good, as did the right one, there was no swelling at all, just twenty stitches waiting to come out. The staff nurse took them out with no trouble whatsoever. Thank God something had gone right at last. So now here I was, ready for some heavy physiotherapy on both legs.

We started in good spirits basking in the sunshine and doing my exercises in a determined manner, with concentration on my quads in both legs, and all was going well. It

148

was hours of 'tighten, relax, tighten, relax', then leg raising of first one leg and then the other. I was always glad though when the exercises were over and I could get back to the safety of the splints and bandages, for any movement of either knee joint caused me severe pain.

Then came the day I had been dreading. My physiotherapist and Sister took off my bandages and splints, and Sister said, 'Knee bending time Raymond.' I knew it had to be done so I said, 'OK let's get on with it then.'

We started on my right leg with just gentle pressure to force my leg up the bed to bend the knee. It was agony. Pain shot up and down my leg. So we eased the leg flat once more, a little rest and then we tried again. But it was no use; even the slightest bend was unbearable. I was willing to keep trying but Sister called a halt and moved onto my left leg and tried to bend that one. It moved enough to allow the passage of Sister's flat hand under my leg, but once again the pain was unbearable and the knee locked tight. So there I was with two very painful knees that wouldn't bend. I was devastated, and it showed, so they called it enough for the session and I wasn't sorry. As they bandaged me back into the safety of my splints and bandages Sister said, 'We will leave you now Raymond – you have enough pain to contend with, and I will see the doctors about you.' The physiotherapist asked me to carry on if possible, with my quads exercises for both legs, as often as I could, which I did, if only gently. The words 'tighten, relax, tighten, relax' were imprinted on my brain. Even this gentle exercise caused serious pain in the joints and I began to have doubts that my legs would ever bend again. My hopes hit rock bottom.

The next day I had numerous visitors, the registrar, Sister, the senior physiotherapist and my own physiotherapist. Both my legs were stripped of the bandages and splints. We then went through the procedure of trying to bend the knees, but there was nothing, only pain. Even my quads were not responding to the exercises. In fact, the whole thing was a total disaster.

My own consultant was away on holiday, so the senior consultant, a professor, the top man at the MRI, came to see me. He arrived with the registrar, Sister and physiotherapists, plus numerous young doctors. I had already had my knees bared for all to see so I lay back and tried to listen to the whispered words being spoken at the end of my bed, it was all about me, but not to me. Then at last they approached my bedside. The consultant asked me first to bend my right leg and then my left, and tighten the quadriceps in both legs, which I tried with little success. It was then that I heard the most unbelievable words from a doctor that I was ever going to hear.

He said, 'Mr Hill, if a good fairy could grant you a wish, which leg would you like to keep?' I was astounded, and I wasn't on my own.

I replied stonily, 'I want to keep both of them, thank you very much.' I was not at all impressed with him. He shook his head and they all moved away.

To say I was seething mad was a serious understatement, and when they had all left the ward Sister came to see me. She could see that I was in a rage. 'Now calm down Raymond, it is only his opinion.'

'But he is supposed to be the best there is, good fairy indeed! The man is a bloody nutter!'

'Oh no he isn't, he is only facing facts Raymond. Unless we make some progress with your legs, something will have to be done.'

'Such as what? What else can we do?' I asked.

'Well to start with, you are going to have two hydrocortisone injections, one in each knee, to try and relieve the pain.' My memories of cortisone injections were not pleasant ones.

'Who is going to do it?'

'Your own registrar.'

'Thank God for small mercies,' I said.

The following day was 20 June, my fortieth birthday. I saw the registrar come into the ward and head in my direction.

'Has Sister told you what's going to happen Raymond?' I nodded my head and tried a brave smile. 'I will do it in the treatment room, not in the ward.' I was grateful for that for I could cry out if I needed to, and I was sure I would. Two nurses wheeled my bed into the anteroom where the doctor and Sister were waiting. Unfortunately I had started with a migraine a few minutes earlier so I couldn't stand the treatment room lights and kept my eyes tightly shut.

'Sister, you will have to hold my legs tightly or else I will move them.'

'Alright, if that is what you want, and I promise you we will be as quick as we can, won't we Doctor?'

'You can bet your life on that, Raymond, it's nearly my coffee break!' He was as good as his word; he first injected the left knee, and then quickly moved on to the right one. The first one was bad enough, but the second was agony, and I was as sick as a dog. I heaved my heart up and couldn't stop. This was partly from the pain, but also from the migraine, so rather than take me back to the ward, they left me where I was in peace and quiet. They put a damp cloth over my eyes to keep out the light and left me to sleep. I stayed there for the rest of the day.

Then, in the very early hours of the following morning as I still lay in the now darkened room where I had been left for the night, I heard the sound of someone entering. Before I had time to think what was happening, a hand was gently but firmly pressing on my face, held so that I couldn't turn to see who it was. Then, incredibly, a hand went down the inside of my shorts, found my 'manhood', and, in what seemed only seconds, it was over. A voice quietly whispered, 'Happy Birthday Raymond' and was gone. As I turned, all I saw in the darkness was a nurse's navy cloak as it vanished through the door. This was surely taking tender loving care to the very extreme. In all the time I was to remain in Crewe ward it was our secret. Mine and a nurse's, who I obviously must have known, but she was determined that I would never know which. And in this, she succeeded.

Then followed weeks of treatment in the physiotherapy

151

department where I was taken in a wheelchair to submit my legs to all kinds of treatments. We had weights, springs, faradism, ultrasonic and ice packs. The right leg was responding slowly to the treatment, both in muscle development and knee bending. It was bloody hard work but we were winning. The left leg on the other hand, was another story. It seemed to be getting worse not better, the knee joint was locked solid with severe adhesions and my quadriceps seemed to be wasting away. There was no strength in the leg at all and it was very disappointing. It had been two months now since the operation on my left leg, two months and I hadn't yet stood on my legs. I was still struggling out of the bed into a wheelchair, then out of the wheelchair onto the plinth for further treatments.

Things weren't bad all the time because I was now also having hydrotherapy and this was the highlight of the treatment. I was pushed over to the pool in my bed, where I had all my bandages removed and my shorts exchanged for my swimming trunks. I was then helped onto a stretcher hoist, and lowered into the water where I was helped off the hoist by two lovely physiotherapists, who exercised me in the water, which was relaxing and warm. I found it unbelievable what I could achieve in the water as opposed to out and dry. After my water treatment I was helped back onto the hoist and lifted up and out. I was then dried and re-bandaged and helped back into bed, then I was returned to the ward or the rose garden.

My right leg was getting stronger every day and so at last I was let out of bed and graduated to the wheelchair to get myself about. I was overjoyed, it felt great! The right leg was left unbandaged and free but the left one was still in its cocoon of splint and bandages so that it stuck out in front of the chair, but I didn't care, I was free of my bed at last. I was independent.

Needless to say, the first place I made for was the loo. It was heavenly bliss to hop my way into the toilet and perch myself on the seat, and not to have to cry for help. I wheeled myself everywhere, I was able to tour the hospital in my own time, and that was something I had a lot of, for apart from the daily and sometimes twice daily trips to the physiotherapist, I was my own man. One place I liked to go was to see the old folks (I don't like the word 'geriatrics') both in the wards and at occupational therapy. I brought out all my old clean jokes and enjoyed seeing them laugh and be happy.

Still the weeks rolled by, with rapid improvement of the right leg and continuous slow grind with the left. I had now graduated to walking between the bars in the gym, facing the mirror to make sure you were walking straight and upright. There was a funny thing with this exercise for at each end of the bars there were mirrors, and for the first time I could see not only my tanned front, but also my snow white back. It certainly looked very odd. I was also having a daily ride on the stationary cycle in the department, I could almost pedal like normal with my right leg, it caused some discomfort but at least I could do it. With the left leg though it was too much to do, I could get the knee partly bent but never a full turn.

By this time three months had passed and I could now take myself to the pool every day. I could change and get myself into the pool by hopping on my now good right leg, which wasn't bad for a leg I was told would only be of 75 to 80 per cent use to me. I could get myself down the steps and then I could swim about by myself. These were some of my happiest moments at Oswestry.

One day, I was in the garden in brilliant sunshine having ice packs on my left knee. I was tanned, wearing sunglasses, smoking a cigar and drinking some iced water, it was more like a holiday than a hospital. It was then that I received a visitor from work. He was a friend of mine who had been working in Holland and he was bringing me some Dutch cigars. He couldn't believe it when he saw me and my physiotherapist. 'Bloody hell, and I have come to see you because I am told you are not very well. You wait 'til I get back to the office!'

Then came the time that I blotted my copy book with my

wheelchair. A few of us that were mobile used to go to the hospital visitors' canteen, which was also the hospital 'tuck shop', to do the shopping for the bedfast lads. It was, more often than not, a race to see who could get there first; we used to dash out of the ward onto the corridor, and wheel like mad to reach the door, which led to a short passage. This, in turn, took you out into the grounds at the rear of the hospital. I used to charge along with my leg stuck out in front like a battering ram, scattering all and sundry. Near the end of the journey there was a slope to be negotiated and a road to cross. For me, on this fateful trip it was to be extremely embarrassing.

I negotiated the slope at full speed, that is until I saw the ambulance approaching on the road. I tried to stop as quickly as I could, nearly breaking my fingers in the process, but I managed to stop the chair. This was fine except that I kept going, and slid out of my seat and finished up in the road, on a very painful backside, right in front of the ambulance which had stopped quite easily when the driver saw me coming. Everyone rushed to my assistance, the driver, nurses, physios and even some visitors. As I lay sprawled on the floor I felt humiliated and wished the ground would open up and swallow me. As the ambulance driver and some nurses lifted me back into my chair, they made sure I was all right, and apart from a bruised backside, all I had was a very damaged ego. I wheeled myself away and back towards my ward with their laughter still ringing in my ears. As I entered the ward I knew that the news of my demise had gone ahead of me and I felt a right bloody fool, that was for sure. Sister came and examined me to make sure I was not hurt at all and apart from a few bruises I was fine. When she was sure that I was all right she read me the riot act and threatened to take my wheelchair off me. Whether it was coincidence or not I don't know, but the next day I was given a pair of elbow crutches in exchange for my chair.

Now this indeed was progress. I think at last I was beginning to see the chance of getting home was much

154

nearer, for I had now been in hospital for three months and it felt like a long time. I was very mobile on my crutches and I could move along at a very fast rate around the grounds. I used to visit everyone I could, especially the old folk in the wards and at occupational therapy, as I used to do in my chair. The story about me falling out of the chair brought many tears of joy. There was one time though when the tears were mine, real tears.

I was unable to do much cycling in the gym for my left leg was still virtually immovable, and my quads were still very weak, it was only this that was keeping me in Oswestry. One day in the occupational therapy department I got on their bike, it was geared up to drive a saw blade on a jig saw. It was used to cut thin sheets of plywood to make jigsaw puzzles. So there I was, barely turning the wheels to work the thing, with the right leg doing all the work as usual, but they all cheered me on. I felt that I had achieved something and made some progress, that is until a small boy of about eight or nine jumped on the saddle and started to pedal. The saw went as if driven by a steam engine. I was heartbroken and I left without a word to anyone, and as I made my way back to the ward there were tears of disappointment in my eyes.

I wasn't down for very long because that Saturday was the Gala Open day for the hospital and all the wards had to enter a bed decorated for the procession. Crewe ward entered my bed, and made it into a cage with cot sides. I was going to be 'Brumas' the giant panda, and one of the other lads was going to be 'Che-Che' my reluctant mate. They bandaged our hands and painted claws on them, but the final thing was the animal heads. They were made out of plaster in the fracture clinic and were excellent but very heavy to wear. We had mouth and eye holes so we could breathe and see what was going on. Frank Bough, whose wife had been a physiotherapist at the hospital, was one of the judges.

The day was boiling hot with the sun beating down; it was a perfect day. That is unless you were wearing a heavy

155

bear's head – we were roasted as we were pushed around the grounds. Needless to say, the kids' ward won, and rightly so, but we were quite well placed. As soon as it was over we took off our panda heads to get some fresh air, but as we did this we heard a little girl burst out crying and we turned to see her sobbing in her mother's arms. 'We have followed you all afternoon and she really thought you were pandas,' the mother explained. By this time we were disrobed completely and the poor girl was still heartbroken as her mother carried her away.

On the following Monday morning, Sister said she hoped that I would be allowed home very soon, as she thought I would most likely continue having treatment for the left leg at the MRI. She said it would all depend on the consultant when he came the following week. I couldn't wait. On the day he was to come I had my wash and shave very early. As I shaved, I realised how well I looked, for my head, face and chest were really very tanned and I looked as if I had been on holiday for almost four months, and not a patient in hospital for that length of time.

The ward round started, and I waited impatiently for them to reach my bed. I sat up very straight and tried to look as fit as a fiddle, which wasn't too hard. Apart from my left leg and its numerous problems, I really did feel better than I had been for years, and all the skin they could see was golden brown. My consultant arrived and stared at me, shook his head and then had a long conversation with the registrar whilst Sister took off my bandages and splint so that he could see the left leg in all its glory. There were hardly any quadriceps to see at all, because despite all the hard work, we were making no progress whatsoever. The consultant felt the quads and tried to bend the knee, but he found it to be stiff and painful.

'How long has he been with you now Sister?'

'Fifteen weeks we have had to suffer,' she replied.

'Well I think that is long enough to be away from home, make arrangements for him to go next week, and I will arrange for his treatment to be carried on at the MRI. Is that all right with you, Mr Hill? Although, I must say you don't look bad to me, you should have had to pay a lot of money for a tan like that.'

The registrar chipped in and said, 'He has spent all this time trying to get a tan as good as mine, but . . .' and before I knew what he was doing, he reached across and tugged my shorts partly down, and showed everyone a snow-white bum '. . . his tan isn't all over like mine is!' I didn't care that everyone was laughing at me, I was overjoyed that I was going home the following week. We had one more week working on the leg and then it was time to go.

Now, sixteen weeks is a long time in hospital, to be nursed, bathed and cared for by the nurses and physiotherapists. You also become very hospitalised with your daily living all planned for you. You just follow the routine and fit in as best you can, until eventually you also become a part of the system. Good treatment and sleep are all part of the hospital way of life. I made my rounds of farewells to various groups of people with whom I had shared my time at Oswestry. I was to go all the way home by ambulance, and it came to collect me from the ward. There were tears from physiotherapists and nurses, and I think even Sister and the registrar had damp eyes. As for myself, I was feeling heartbroken, it was really great to be going home, but it was also sad to be leaving my home of the last four months.

So that was the end of an era, now it was back to the MRI.

21

The first day after I arrived home there was a knock on the door at 8.30 a.m. It was the ambulance ready to take me to the hospital for treatment. Talk about 'no rest for the wicked'.

The Head of the physiotherapy department saw me on arrival. He examined the leg and took some measurements of my quadriceps.

'Well, Mr Hill, we have a mountain to climb here, but rest assured, with your help we will win.' Who the hell was he kidding? It certainly wasn't me. My left knee was solid now, and my quadriceps virtually non-existent, and I had bloody well worked hard in Oswestry.

Three times a week we tried every trick in the book, we went through weights, springs, faradism, ultrasonic, hot towels and ice packs, plus every exercise in the book. They got the knee to bend slightly but it caused intense pain. Then after three months as an out-patient we reached the walking stage without my crutches and without the support of the splint and bandages, but holding onto the bars in the gym. I must admit that I was always very reluctant to move without the safety of my 'Thompson splint' and bandages. I was always scared that my legs would not support me as I walked, and on more than one occasion this was the truth, and I would fall into the physiotherapist's arms a disappointed and disgusted man.

After another four weeks of trailing backwards and forwards as an out-patient, I was seen by the consultant. I think he was as disappointed as I was. The physiotherapists told him that even with my high pain threshold they could make little or no progress with my quadriceps, that they had been able to bend it, but only very painfully – for me, not them. So it was decided that I would have to have another operation on the left leg.

'Jesus Christ, not another,' I mumbled.

'I am sorry but we will have to do a placation of your quads to make them shorter. That will give them more strength to hold your leg straight and firm, and it will also help your bending.'

Expecting weeks of waiting, I was surprised when they told me it would be done the following week in the MRI, and that they would need me to go into the hospital on Sunday. I thought, wait until I tell them at home. As I was being pushed back to the physiotherapy department after having seen the consultant, there was just one question I wanted answered.

'What do you mean when you say that I have a high pain threshold? I haven't heard of that before.' It was explained to me that people have a high or low pain threshold, but that mine was very high, and that being so, I could stand a lot more pain than most, as I had been doing for almost the past year. Yes, it was almost a year since my operation on the left leg. The right leg, which I had been told would only be a 75 to 80 per cent good leg, was reacting wonderfully well to all the extra pressure that had been put on it in the last few months. I decided that from then on my pain threshold was definitely going to go down a few notches.

My operation was on 4 May, 1970.

I had gone in and been through the routine, until the arrival of the operation day. I had my leg shaved and painted again, and then sheeted up and made ready for the theatre. I had been told that I was the last on the list for the day, so there I lay in my back to front night-shirt. As I watched patients go and then come back to the ward, I thought how much better this system was than the one at Oswestry.

It was about two o'clock when Sister came to give me my

159

pre-med., a quick needle expertly done, in my backside. I had felt so many that I didn't care anymore.

'Now relax Raymond, and go to sleep, you won't be waiting long.' I did exactly as I had been told and went into a deep sleep.

The next thing I heard and felt was the shaking of my bed. It was the staff nurse.

'Thank goodness that's over,' I mumbled drowsily, but then was easily shocked back to being very wide awake.

'What do you mean Raymond? I am just going to take you.' What a disappointment, I just couldn't believe it. I knew it was true for there was the theatre orderly waiting for me with his trolley. It was the beginning of a very familiar journey, looking upwards at the ceiling lights, even the bump as we went into the lift. Then there I was, once again, in the anaesthetist's room for my knock-out drop. One small jab in the back of my hand and a reverse count to four I think, then I was gone.

The next time I opened my eyes again I was back in the ward, curtains around my bed, and as usual heaving my heart up. This time I knew something was different, very different indeed. I had the sickness, I had the pain, but also I had a very heavy leg, which every time I rolled to the side to be sick, tried to drag me back again. I felt around and quickly discovered the reason. Not only had I had the operation, but also the leg was encased in plaster from my thigh down to my ankle. This, they had not told me about. It was heavy and it hurt like hell.

For the next few days I continued to be sick, even though I had injections that were supposed to stop it. I knew that nature would run its course and my sickness would stop when my body wanted it to. And that was on the fourth day. It was a gigantic relief to suddenly find I wasn't sick anymore, the pain from my leg, though, was getting worse and the plaster seemed to hurt more and more. Fortunately for me, the plaster ended at my ankle so that my foot was visible at the bottom of my open cage, where the sheets were folded back to let the air circulate. This gave the chap opposite a perfect view of the bottom of my foot. After three days, he called my wife over to him and told her that he thought my foot was turning black. She informed Sister and . . . bingo! Before I knew where I was, I was back in the fracture clinic where they made one long saw cut along the full length of the plaster. It was not long before I felt the pressure begin to ease in my leg, and my foot began to look its right colour again.

After just a few days I was sent home in an ambulance to once more become an out-patient in the physiotherapy department. It called three times a week to take me back for treatment. There was not a lot we could do with the left leg except for muscle tightening exercises, so most of the time was concentrated on my right leg to keep it strong for the extra work that lay ahead of it. Again.

Five weeks later they took me back to the fracture clinic where I had had my plaster removed. Because they had cut it in such a way, the back of the plaster could act as a long splint. A sister took out my stitches then bandaged me up again, but using the plaster as a support, it made me feel very secure. It was now back to physiotherapy three times a week.

At first it was light quads work and very gentle knee bending, but this was, once again, sheer agony. I felt as though the leg was never ever going to bend again. The operation though, seemed to have been successful as far as my quads were concerned, for slowly but surely my muscles were coming back to life. We did every exercise there was, that is apart from knee bending. I was over the moon that after all this time I could actually see my quadriceps working as they should, it had been a long time, it was well over a year since the removal of my kneecap. But for all the progress we had with the muscles, there was no further improvement with the bending, and what little there was caused me tremendous suffering and pain, and I was always glad to get back to the comfort and safety of my splint.

In spite of all the pain there were always incidents in the department which seemed to ease or lessen the suffering, and we had plenty of laughs, often at the poor physiothera-pist's expense. The time that evoked the most laughter was one day while we were all sat outside, awaiting the arrival of the girls to sort us out into groups or classes, or in my case, individual treatment. Then arrived a girl who was new to all of us. She started to divide us all into our respective classes, when she suddenly announced, 'Sue will take the early leg class, Carol will take the late leg class, and I will take the middle leg class.' The place was in uproar as we all shouted that we wanted to be in her class. The poor lass never lived it down.

I went to see the consultant at regular intervals, always to be told to 'keep up the good work', which we did. We did it three times a week for 24 weeks. Yes, six months. It was now 30 weeks since my last operation, my 'placation', the operation that was going to put me right once and for all. The only real progress we had made was with my quads, they were beginning to work quite well, and I could do all the exercises quite easily. I could do everything except bend the leg more than three inches, and that was a bend that caused very great pain.

At this stage the head of the physiotherapy department said, 'Enough is enough. There is a limit to what you can stand and a limit to what we can do for you.' It was November 1970.

So it was back to the out-patient's clinic, only to find that another of my consultants had moved on to pastures new so I saw the new registrar who examined the leg, especially the knee, and read the physiotherapist's report. He looked through my bulging file and x-rays and said to me quite calmly, 'This sometimes happens to the knee joint after repeated surgery, which you have had in July 1964, May 1969 and May 1970. So what I am saying is, that if we stop treatment for a few months and the leg is still giving you problems, and the worst comes to the worst we can always consider stiffening the leg or even doing an amputation.'

As I got over the shock I asked, 'If you stiffen the leg is it sure to remove the pain?' His answer shook me rigid.

'I very much doubt it.' So that left only one alternative. Amputation.

So here I was, seven months after my operation, with now quite well developed quadriceps, but with very little bend in the leg, and what little bend there was, was extremely painful. How I wished I had never seen a football or cricket ball. I was dissatisfied, disillusioned and disgusted at the whole affair, so I limped out of the hospital with no support on the leg and walking with the aid of a stick.

Painful time passed, with my knee getting steadily more unbearable with each passing day. It was now nearly Christmas 1970 and no amount of medication gave me any relief. It was just a life of constant nagging pain, and there was still no further movement in the knee. None. I was becoming very depressed indeed, I was antisocial at work and I must have been very hard to live with at home. The stage was reached when I thought that all the suffering hadn't been worth it. I could easily have ended it, I had enough tablets to do it, but my family came first. My wife and I knew that I had to do something, so we decided that I would go privately to see the surgeon who had done my first operation, back in July 1964.

So on the 30 December we were off to St. John Street. I went for my consultation with a man for whom I had a great deal of respect, and I was determined that anything that he suggested, I would do, no matter what. It was a very positive attitude but I had suffered more than enough. The surgeon examined me and listened briefly to the history of events. He said that he thought that the placation had to be done, but that it may have been done too tightly, hence the lack of knee movement and the pain. He agreed to take me into hospital for an exploratory operation, which I quickly consented to.

Weeks and months slipped by until March 1971 when I went in for the operation, which was done on 15 March. The pain had steadily increased, with the painful area now reaching down to just below the knee. The exploration, now the fourth operation on the same leg in eight years, showed

163

that the placation sutures on the inside stitching had not dissolved as they should have done, and therefore there were four irregular masses of tough white tissue. Each mass contained black suture material, and these were removed, and the knee thoroughly cleaned up. Almost immediately after the operation some pain had gone, and I could feel that the knee was losing that horrible nagging pain that had been my constant companion for over a year. Ten days went by, then my stitches were removed and the physiotherapy began on the knee. Within a few days we were bending the leg with very little discomfort. I was over the moon. To this day I am convinced that unless that operation had been carried out, I would have lost my leg eventually, and from the pain I had felt, it would not have been in the far distant future.

I now became an out-patient at yet another hospital, but not for long, for within five weeks we had my quads back and my leg bending almost perfectly. As a matter of fact one of my physiotherapists at the MRI was now at this hospital, and she was amazed, more than I was, at my progress. I was wearing no support on the leg and needed just one stick for walking. On discharge, I shook hands with the surgeon who said, 'Well that should be it, you should now have two comparatively good knees, but keep up the exercises constantly.' It was now the end of May, 1971.

Seven years and seven operations, and also years of physiotherapy, and at last I was going to be free of it, or was I?

22

Yet again, my left leg wasn't finished with me. After a few months I was just as bad again, the knee was exceedingly painful in the joint and the area just below it, and it was limiting my movements. Yet on the other hand it would just give in on me without warning.

So, in November 1971 I was back at the hospital as an out-patient. We started with hydrocortisone injections; these had little or no effect, so we went back to giving the knee some support to try and ease the pain and to stop the leg giving way under pressure. The first type of splint was to no avail and it made it difficult for me to do my work correctly. The consultant then decided he would help me by having a calliper made with clips on, which would enable me to bend my knee when I was sitting down. It was a big heavy contraption of leather and steel, with the straps around my ankle, my calf and my thigh. Then it had steel bars down either side of the leg, but with wire clips at the knee to enable me to bend the knee when I wanted to. At first the thing felt like a ton weight, and I was very reluctant to wear it, but I put it on and persevered.

I had been wearing it only a short time, just a matter of a few weeks, when suddenly I became aware of another pain, this time in my left leg near my ankle. By this time I was limping very badly at work and not feeling at all well. Things deteriorated rapidly, and I was taken from work to the doctor's. He examined me quickly and ordered me home to bed.

'You have phlebitis,' he told me. 'Off your feet quickly, and bed rest.' He gave me a prescription to take to the chemist for ointment and tablets. I duly collected these and limped wearily home where I dragged myself upstairs to bed. I painted my ankle with the black substance and took some tablets. It was now early afternoon and I was glad, very glad, to lie back and rest, but it wasn't for long because the pain in the ankle increased, and soon the whole leg felt terrible, right from the ankle to the groin.

The pain continued to increase, and by now I was feeling really ill and wishing that my wife would return. Suddenly, out of the blue there was a new, completely different pain. It was in my chest. At first I just felt the tightness as though my chest was being encircled in a band of steel that was gradually getting tighter and tighter. Breathing was becoming difficult and very painful and I started to roll about the bed to try and alter my position, to ease the terrible pressure, but nothing helped. The pain only became worse and everything began to blur. My eyes couldn't focus properly and I seemed to drift into a coma. I came out of it to find that the pain had increased a hundred-fold, and that I was having to fight for my life. The situation was deteriorating every minute and I seemed to drift in and out of the coma.

Fortunately, by some miracle, my wife arrived home from the shops and heard my frantic efforts to breathe. I had ceased to roll about now and just lay in the coma. One look at me sent her scurrying next door for my neighbour, a St Johns Ambulance Officer. Her arrival on the scene invoked frantic efforts to try and contact my doctor by phone, but this time, of all times, the phone was out of action, so my wife went next door and phoned from there. Fortunately the surgery was quite close, so the doctor ran across the road, came upstairs to look at me, then raced away again, back to the surgery for his bag and to phone for the ambulance. He returned very quickly and gave me an injection. I was now in a deep coma and was not aware of what was happening to me.

The ambulance arrived in minutes and I was immediately given oxygen and then rushed off to the local hospital, I

166

was given oxygen all the way there by the ambulance man. On my arrival at the hospital I was rushed into intensive care and put into an oxygen tent. I had further injections and then I was put onto two drips and then left by the doctors to fight my way through it. It was explained to my wife that I had suffered a major pulmonary embolism, and that blood clots were zooming up my left leg through the groin and then thudding into my body and then going their own way. So my blood was being thinned and then it was up to me.

I remained critically ill for two days and two nights. Then slowly but surely, I regained consciousness and began to look about me and at my surroundings. I was lying very still in the bed with an oxygen mask helping me to breathe, and two drips coming down from suspended bottles, into my arm. I felt terribly weak and still suffered chest pain, but I had survived the crisis. With the help of a devoted hospital staff I was now going to recover. My family was overjoyed but no one as much as I was. I was told they were thinning my blood to prevent further clots developing, and that I would have to rest for a few days or even weeks. After another couple of days in intensive care I was sent upstairs to the ward. I still had my drips attached to me but I was moved with no problem whatsoever.

Time is a great healer and as each day passed, the more I improved, helped by an excellent staff led by a wonderful Sister. She was great; she devoted every minute of her time and her nurses' time to caring for every patient. No one was more important than another. She was very strict but within reason we could laugh and joke with everyone and there was lots of laughter. The more I recovered the more I felt the need to laugh and be happy, for I had been so near to doing neither. So I did my best to bring laughter to the fore with practical jokes, and turning every innocent phrase into a different meaning. Often I went too far and had to be chastised by Sister herself, she knew I meant well so my lectures were nearly all of the gentle variety.

After a couple of weeks I was taken out onto the balcony,

it was great there for even though we were squashed together like sardines in a can, you knew that once you got out there that home was in sight. We were a mixture of patients, from hernias to heart attacks. No matter what the complaint it was everyone's aim to occupy a balcony bed.

I had been on the balcony for about a week when the doctors told me that I could go home. It was brilliant news; I couldn't wait until the family came that night so that I could give them the good news. My companion in the next bed had also been told he was going home so we were both quite excited. He had suffered a large heart attack a few weeks before. We were both full of the joys of spring and couldn't wait to tell our visitors the good news, everyone was laughing and getting very excited, especially my next door neighbour and his friends.

Eventually the bell went to tell the visitors that it was time to go, and we all said our goodbyes as they left the ward. Then the normal procedure was to jump out of bed and watch our visitors move away across the car park. This time though, it was going to be very different, oh how much different! Before we got out of bed, it was a case of 'have you heard this?' and we exchanged jokes that our visitors had told us. I leant across my bed and said, 'Have you heard this silly joke about the Irish Mountain Climbers? What would you call them if they all fell off the mountain?' And before he could answer I told him, 'A Navvylanche!' He burst out laughing very loudly and then he threw his arms skywards and fell towards me. I knew at once that something was drastically wrong, so I dived across and caught him just before his head hit the floor. I was holding onto his shoulders, and at the same time yelling my head off for Sister, a cry taken up by other patients on the balcony when they saw the both of us half hanging out of our beds. The thought crossed my mind, bloody hell, he's heavy! I was straining every muscle so that he wouldn't fall onto the floor.

Suddenly, the balcony was full of people – patients, Sister, nurses and doctors. The weight was taken from my arms

168

and the curtains drawn about the bed, but as I couldn't move from my position I watched in horror at all the efforts being made to save a life that deep down, I knew was already gone. They fought on and on with every trick they knew but the poor fellow was dead. They quietly removed the body from the ward, and then Sister came to draw back the curtains and as she did so, she saw me still hanging half in and half out of bed.

'Raymond stop being so nosy and get back into your bed.' I was more than a little bit upset, for those last few minutes had been, to say the least, very frightening.

'I am not being nosy Sister,' I said testily, 'this is the same position I was in when I caught him, and I can't bloody move.' She was quick to my rescue.

'Oh Raymond, I am sorry but I didn't realise your predicament.' She shouted for help, and with the assistance of two nurses, they got me back in bed. It was exceedingly painful, but after what had gone on before, I clenched my teeth and didn't cry out. They removed my pillows so that I was perfectly flat, in agony, and as usual my left leg was killing me. Fortunately for me there was an orthopaedic consultant in the hospital visiting other patients so he came along to see me. As he came to the bed we were both surprised, as we knew each other slightly.

'Hello Mr Hill, what have you been doing to yourself?' Sister explained the situation to him and he nodded his head and said, 'Well let me have a look at him then.' It wasn't a long look and I didn't have to move myself, he just lifted my leg and watched my face change colour.

'I think you have slipped a disc, so we will take the necessary precautions. A board please Sister, and two weeks as he is now.'

I was dumfounded.

'But I am supposed to be going home in the morning.'

He shook his head.

'I am afraid not, and I will see you tomorrow.' And away he went. I stared at Sister, still in deep shock. 'I don't believe that this is really happening to me.' I was near to tears of frustration.

'I am going to give you an injection to ease the pain, then I suggest that you rest quietly until we bring the board to slide under your mattress. And don't worry, I will phone Mrs Hill and tell her of your predicament.'

I had to smile as I said, 'She will only see the funny side of it if I know her,' which I believe she did.

As for the ward, life had to go on as normal, so my board was brought and eased carefully under my mattress. As I stared up at the ceiling I thought of the change in just two short hours since the end of visiting time at eight o'clock. My problem seemed insignificant compared to the death of my companion, and with that thought I drifted off to sleep.

Days went by, and apart from my bad leg and back I was now fine, but I was bored with just staring up at the ceiling. So I began to be a bit of a playful nuisance to the nurses and the physiotherapists who now visited me (I couldn't seem to get away from those girls!). One of my favourite tricks on a new young nurse was to put anything I could into my urine bottle, anything from orange juice, lemonade or lemon and barley. They could always get their own back though, as I now had to depend on help to use a bed pan, and there was many an occasion that they helped me to balance on a very warm pan.

The two weeks of bed rest passed by, and I had another visit from the surgeon. He lifted my legs one at a time, but there was still a lot of pain with the lifting of the leg.

'I think another week Sister, but the physiotherapists can show him how to sit up straight for meal times.' It was not what I had expected but at least it was progress of a sort. The following morning my physiotherapist arrived to teach me how to roll over on my side and push myself up sideways into a sitting position. Everything was fine other than my painful left leg. I often wondered if I should have had it taken off when I had the chance, at least it wouldn't hurt then.

It was then that I started to have trouble with my tongue

170

and throat and even the roof of my mouth. It was all a mess and I had to have my mouth swabbed three times a day. It wasn't painful as such, but it was another setback and it worried me, and it seemed to worry Sister for she often swabbed me herself. I had still stayed out on the balcony all the time since the calamity.

Then one night at visiting time, Sister came along to me with my file and a swab dish in her hands. She asked my visitors to leave for a few minutes as an Ear, Nose and Throat Specialist was coming to look at my mouth. She carefully laid the file and swab dish on my bed and then removed my glasses. Now, without them I couldn't see any faces clearly and in fact I had to wear my glasses to shave, with. By this time my back had improved so much that I was now sat up with three pillows behind me, which Sister now removed and made me lie down flat.

'This is a bit unfair at visiting time Sister, couldn't he come at any other time?'

Her reply was, 'Don't be cheeky,' then she went away. So there I was, lying flat on my back and staring at the ceiling. My wife popped her head in and said that she would wait outside until the doctor had been. To say that I was worried was putting it mildly, I was really scared. What else could go wrong? I was sweating pints and my pyjamas were soon soaked. I then heard a foreign voice talking to my wife and Sister outside the curtains and thought, oh God what is wrong with me? Eventually the doctor and Sister came through the curtains to examine me. I could just about make out that Sister had given the doctor a swab from the spatula dish. A foreign voice told me to open my mouth and stick out my tongue. He kept repeating to himself 'Ja, ja, ja' as he swabbed my mouth, throat and tongue. By this time I was saturated with perspiration, it poured from my head and under my armpits; I was in a hell of a state. The Sister and doctor went into a huddle and called my wife in.

After a little while he came over to me and said, in broken English, 'I am very sorry Mr Hill, but your tongue will have to come out. I am going to have to cut it off!' I

171

was astounded, but only then did I hear the giggles coming from the other patients and their visitors. The Sister gave me back my glasses, and pulled the curtains back to reveal everyone trying to restrain their mirth. All the nurses were at the end of the ward, also laughing.

Sister said to me, 'That serves you right Raymond, you have had this coming for a long time.' What had happened was that the so-called German was a patient who, when he was in the hospital, had suffered some of my jokes. He had phoned Irene, my wife, and the Sister to see if I was well enough to have a practical joke played on me for a change. Both parties were all for it and my mouth infection gave them the real opportunity, as already my wife and the Sister knew that it was thrush. This was the second time I had suffered from that in my hospital career.

At last I was ready for home, fit again after seven weeks in hospital. All I had to do was to continue to wear a pair of white elasticated thrombosis stockings, and to treat my back gently for a few more weeks. And most of all, not to wear the calliper again. So yet again I became an out-patient, twice a week to the physiotherapy department and once weekly to the anticoagulant clinic. This was to last for about twelve months or so, and the only thing they couldn't cure was my bad left leg but that didn't seem so important now. I was fairly fit again and playing hard. I gave up football management and the inclement weather that went with it, and took up Scouting as my leisure activity.

23

The years rolled by until the summer of 1980, and whilst on a tour of Holland with the Scout and Guide Band, I became very ill and collapsed halfway through the tour with apparent exhaustion. A severe pain in my upper back, just between my shoulder blades accompanied this. On my return to England a few days later I seemed to perk up again, but I could do nothing to alleviate the pain in my back. My doctor at first thought it was a worsening of my lower back problem from the disc trouble, for I was often troubled by that. But he decided that I needed to be seen by a specialist at the hospital for I was now losing weight rapidly. I had to stop wearing my rings as they just slipped off my fingers, my watch slid down over my wrist, and I had to pull my belt in a few holes to keep my trousers up.

It was just a few weeks to wait but in that short time I had still been losing weight, and the pain in the back had increased. When I looked at myself in the mirror, my face had become drawn and I was very worried, but I tried not to show it to my family. At the hospital I was examined and questioned about all my symptoms, and it was decided that I would have to go into the hospital for a couple for days for further tests, and that was going to be the very next day.

I was in hospital for a few days at first for the tests, every orifice in my body had something pushed into it, and in between I had complete bed rest. I had special x-rays of my kidneys and liver, still with no definite reasons for my pain and exhaustion. By this time I think that more than a little depression was setting in, so they sent me home for the weekend to cheer me up. On my return the consultant told me that he wasn't quite sure what was wrong with me and that I was going to be sent to other hospitals for more tests. The first one was in Withington; here I was to have a tube down my throat under anaesthetic. This was a failure because they couldn't get the tube down, no matter how hard they tried. I was allowed to rest for a few days and then I was sent to Manchester Royal Infirmary for a full bone scan, once more a special dye was injected into my arm, then after a short rest the scan was carried out. This again with negative results. So off I went, back to A6 at Stepping Hill Hospital.

Through all this doubt and strain I was nursed by the most wonderful Irish Sister who kept my spirits up and didn't let me get too depressed, to her I will always be eternally grateful. I wasn't as perky as usual, but my glib tongue still got me into trouble on the odd occasion.

After about three more weeks, it was decided that I could have something wrong with my pancreas, and that I was going to the Medical School in Manchester University for one more, final test. Getting there was like a scene from a *Carry On* film. I was accompanied by a nurse from the ward and we were sent by taxi. Now, the driver didn't know how to get to the rear ambulance entrance, so he dropped us, in the morning rush hour, on the main road facing the school. So there we were, my nurse and I stranded on the wrong side of the road, me in my pyjamas and dressing gown, and my poor nurse with no coat or cloak. We really looked out of place trying to cross the road at that time in the morning. Eventually the problem was solved by a couple of kind car drivers who saw our predicament and halted to let us cross. I know that I felt really stupid as we made our way over the road and up the wide steps leading into the building. With the help of a kindly porter's directions we were able to find the people we needed.

I was taken to a cubicle where I took off my dressing gown and my pyjama top. Then, clad only in my pyjama trousers, I made my way into a large room where the CAT scan machine was located. It was here that I was given yet another injection by a lady doctor, who then explained briefly what was going to happen to me once the dye had circulated. All I had to do was to climb aboard the machine, which resembled a torpedo tube cut in half, she would then leave me alone whilst the machine was doing its work. She stressed that though I might feel sick, they would like me to try very hard not to be. I promised to do my best for them. She helped me to board the machine and get settled into a comfortable lying position, and then after asking me to lie as still as possible, she left the room and joined the others behind a glass screen. I was very apprehensive, but at the same time very conscious of how lucky I was to have all these people who were at the very top of their profession looking after me. It was soon over and I said my goodbyes and we went back to the hospital, this time in a taxi whose driver knew his directions well. There was a strange incident in the journey which was when the driver, who was very friendly, looked at me in his mirror and said that he hoped I wouldn't mind him saying that he thought I looked far too well to be in hospital. This was apparently the effect of the injection, which gave my skin a kind of golden glow for a while.

On my return to Stepping Hill I was glad to climb into bed for a rest and a little nap. My sojourn was disturbed by the arrival of my consultant and the Sister. I knew instantly that something was seriously wrong with me. Sister pulled the curtains around the bed and he sat on it.

'I am afraid, Mr Hill, that I have some very bad news for you. All of our tests so far prove that you have three tumours on your pancreas. In plain English Mr Hill, you have cancer.'

I looked at them both and said, 'I thought by now that it was going to be something like that.' I was surprised at my matter of fact voice, and my seemingly instant acceptance of the blow.

'All your symptoms, pain for so long, loss of weight, listlessness are all things that convince us, and this is what your last test on the 'CAT scan' machine has proved. But even now I want you to be seen by one more specialist, will you do that for me?' I nodded my head, what had I got to lose?

'Yes certainly I will, when and where?'

'Tonight after visiting, he will come to the ward to see you. Sister will bring him to you later.'

She then spoke for the first time. 'We will be seeing your wife tonight Raymond, before visiting.'

'Has she any idea yet, or not?' I asked.

The consultant said, 'I think she obviously knows by seeing the change in you that something is very seriously wrong with you.' It was only then that it hit me. What was going to happen to Irene and my sons? How was I going to face up to them?

As they were going away Sister asked, 'Do you want to be left quietly like this, or shall I draw the curtains back for you?'

'No Sister, please leave them together for now whilst I have a quiet think to myself.' They left me to my thoughts. What they had said didn't really surprise me, but now that it seemed definite I had some serious thinking to do, and four serious questions to ask myself. How do I face it? What do I do about it? How long will it last? Do I let them operate or not? Or lastly the additional forlorn question, or shall I drown myself in the bathroom? As the questions and answers were milling about in my brain, I had another visitor. It was the medical consultant that they had told me was coming later.

'Hello Mr Hill, I have been asked to give you a quick once over, do you mind?' So I went through another routine but thorough check up. He asked lots of questions and I gave loads of honest answers.

'OK Mr Hill, that's all I can do for you, so goodnight.' And a goodnight to you, I thought. After a while I got out of bed and pulled the curtains back, I was composed and ready to face the world, but first of all was the family.

The very next day we had another problem with the left leg, this time it was a deep vein thrombosis. It was extremely painful but they soon had me sorted out, and before I knew where I was, I was on the drip again and being given the once over by the ECG (echocardiogram) unit daily.

My wife and the doctors had a meeting at which every aspect of the case was gone over carefully between them. They all agreed that there should not be an operation, that I had been through enough already and it would be better to leave things as they were, and that decision was passed on to me. They may have agreed between themselves, but in the end it was for me to decide, and me alone. I was the one with all the pain and with a responsibility to my wife and sons, and I needed to know for sure how long I had got. My thrombosis was now in check with Warfarin tablets and I was off the drip, so it was decided that I could go home for a few days for a change. I think deep down they kept hoping that I would get fed up with it all and decide to stay at home and not go back.

It was whilst I was at home that I planned a whole new kitchen and dining area, and this was going to be done immediately by a friend. So I easily got a second mortgage to pay for it, knowing that it would only be short term because very soon my pension would take care of my expenses. I had now completely come to terms with myself and I knew what I must do. It wasn't what the surgeon or my wife wanted but in the end it was my life, and also by this time I was getting weaker and I was in more pain. Then to top it all I discovered another area of intense pain. It was my left groin. My own GP examined me and told me that I had yet another hernia and this time it was a bad one. I felt that this was the least of my worries, but I did promise him that I would tell the hospital when I went back.

My period of grace out of hospital came to an end and off I went back to my favourite Irish sister in A6 who ushered me into the first bed on the left-hand side. No sooner had I got in bed when the ward round started. I was the first on the agenda.

'Hello Mr Hill, have you enjoyed your few days at home?'

177

I told him that I had, and then I told him about the hernia. He examined me and agreed that it was indeed a bad one.

'What am I going to do with you Mr Hill?' It was my turn now.

'Well Sir, I want the operation as soon as you can do it, and I don't mean the operation for the hernia, I mean the big one. It is important to me to know how long I have got, I really need to know for there are plans that have to be made.'

'Raymond, none of us want you to have it, not even your wife.' He was not happy.

'I am sorry, but I say yes!' He appeared to give in.

'Alright, I will operate, but not yet, there is your thrombosis problem and also now the hernia to be repaired. I will not operate until I am satisfied that all is well for both of us, it will be Friday at the earliest.' He shook his head and then went into deep conversation with the Sister and house doctor. I couldn't hear, it must have been about me but at least I had got my own way.

For the rest of the week I had more blood taken and numerous injections fired back in again. The ECG people were constantly at my bedside, everyone was giving me their best attention. Thursday night's visiting was a quiet one for us, all the family was against my decision but I knew it had to be. It turned out to be a tearful goodbye as the bell called an end to visiting.

After the visitors had gone and the supper drinks had been served I had two more visitors, the consultant and the anaesthetist. The consultant sat and waited whilst I was examined and passed as fit for the operation. It was then that I was asked yet again by him, 'Do you still want to go ahead with this?'

'Yes Sir, that I do,' I replied.

'Well then we go ahead with the operation in the morning, and depending on the results of that I may do the hernia at the same time, we will have to see how it goes.' We shook hands as he got up to go.

'Thanks,' was all I could say.

178

I passed a fairly good night with the aid of two sleeping-pills, but I was awake very early, about five o'clock, and had no sooner sat up in bed when the night Sister came round. She asked me again if I wanted to go ahead with the operation, or had I had a change of mind.

'No Sister, I need to know for sure.'

She left me with a kind, 'Good luck then Raymond.' It was, as usual, no food or drink, and on the top of my bed was clipped the 'Nil by Mouth' notice. It needn't have been there because I couldn't have swallowed anything anyway, I was thinking too much of what lay ahead of me this day. The day staff came on duty so my night nurses left me with a kiss for good luck. As soon as breakfast was over and the day's duties began, Sister came to see me and she also asked me if I still wanted to go ahead with everything.

'Yes Sister, my mind is definitely made up, I am sure I am doing the right thing, but thanks for asking.' She cared for her patients, that was for sure.

It wasn't long before a theatre orderly came through to shave me. My neck down to my groin was cleared of hair and I then went for a bath. As I lay there soaking in a very full bath I was meditating on the day's coming events. I thought how easy it would be to gently slide under the water and end it all. That thought was soon dispelled for I thought of my wife and sons, and all the people in the hospital who were trying to make me well again. I climbed out just as a nurse came for me.

'Come on Raymond, we are going to get you ready, it is nearly time.' I put on my 'back to front nightie' yet again, and made my way back to my bed. Sister was there with my pre-med needle, which she gently gave me in my backside.

'Now relax and try to have a sleep.' Well, I did drop off and I was awakened by the arrival of the theatre trolley. I was soon on it and wheeled away very quietly. That seemed strange as there were no shouts of good luck or any call of encouragement, but as nearly all of them knew the situation, they were, I think, inwardly wishing me luck.

It was only a short journey from A6 to the operating

179

theatre and the anaesthetist's room where the surgeon met me.

'Good Morning Mr Hill, are you all ready for this?' I nodded my answer and he went on, 'We will play it by ear, if the first operation only takes a short time I will repair your hernia as well.' I thought it was good value, two for the price of one! The anaesthetist soon put me to sleep; I didn't even have time to count. The next thing I remembered was being told to 'wake up, wake up!'. Then through my muddled brain I could hear some kind of rattling noise; I couldn't make it out but after more cries of 'wake up, wake up!' I forced my eyes open. The surgeon was kneeling by the side of my bed, he was still in his green theatre gear and he was rattling something in his hand. I could see his lips moving but at first I couldn't make out the words, then after a few minutes they came through the fog. He was shouting in an excited voice, 'no cancer, no cancer!' I immediately dropped off into a deep sleep.

The next thing that awakened me was pain, my chest and stomach were killing me, so I opened my eyes and felt about me. I first felt around my groin and could feel no dressing so I thought that they hadn't done it because they had found cancer. I felt dreadful. I was hot and in real, real pain, and as usual I felt, and was, sick. I tried hard not to heave because that brought me intense pain in my chest. At last I looked down at my chest and stomach. I was astounded. I could see a cut that seemed enormous and I seemed to be being held together by four very large stitches, as well as many normal ones. I seemed to have tubes everywhere – my nose, stomach and my hand. I looked and felt dreadful. The thought occurred to me that this was the beginning of the end.

I was soon spotted by the alert nursing staff as now being awake and one of them came to help me as I struggled to lift myself to be sick, whilst another one went to fetch Sister. Now I would get to know the worst. But as she approached my bed she was all smiles and very perky, I just couldn't understand her attitude, for I felt very far from smiling, that

I can assure you. Before she said anything, she took a small plastic container off my locker and rattled it repeatedly. I knew I had heard that sound before, but where? Her face had a smile a mile wide.

'Good news Raymond, very good news, there is no cancer. Do you hear? No cancer!' And then I remembered where I had heard that sound before. 'The doctors are thrilled to bits, I believe that they were cheering in the theatre.'

She then sat on my bed, held my hand and explained that my gall bladder with large stones had enveloped my pancreas, and the stones in every test had shown to be tumours. At the same time they were not allowing my pancreas to function properly, hence all my weight loss and pain. She was so excited that I couldn't get a word in, but even she had to stop for a second breath and I got in quickly with the most important question of all.

'Does Irene know?' I asked.

She nodded her head vigorously, 'Yes, he phoned her immediately after he came to see you.'

The news was marvellous for everyone, especially me, for it was all over. I looked down at myself in disbelief, I didn't care how big the stitches or how many there were, or even how bad I felt at that moment. All I knew was that I could only get better from now on. It didn't matter how hard it was going to be, now I knew that I was going to survive.

It was at this time of my gradual recovery that my hospital world was shattered. My wonderful Irish Sister on A6, who was mainly responsible, with her nursing staff for this recovery, had told her friend that I was in A6. This friend was the Sister who had cared for me back in traumatic 1973 on B3 ward. We had so much laughter together! She sent me a message that she would come and see me the next morning when she came off duty. By now, I was on the balcony, always a sign that things were going well. Morning arrived with me to meet this wonderful angel again. Hours went by and no one came to see me, no one, no Sister, no nurses, no doctor, no one. I just couldn't understand it.

181

Then, just before lunch I had a visitor at last, a young house doctor. That something was wrong was very obvious, for he was certainly unhappy with his task. The blow, when he eventually managed to tell me, was heartbreaking. My lovely Sister had collapsed and died on her own ward that morning before she was due to come to see me.

God, if you are there, where is your justice?

Once again, I obeyed all the rules and concentrated on my recovery and three weeks later I was allowed home yet again. Then began a long return to fitness, and once again I was an out-patient, this time at the anticoagulant clinic for the next twelve months.

24

The hospital allowed me exactly that time to completely recover then they sent for me again, this time to repair my hernia. It should have been quite simple but it wasn't.

My consultant though, did another superb job on what turned out to be a double tear, even though it meant losing my left testicle before it could do me any harm. I was hospitalised for another four weeks, due mainly to the fact that I had thrombosis in my left leg yet again. It seemed that just a few days in bed were enough for this problem to return, so once again I was on the drip to thin my blood, and this was followed by regular Hefrin injection into the stomach. This was an injection few of the nurses liked giving for some reason. Once again I was wearing my white stockings, these were fine when you had to stay in bed, but once you were up and about they were always coming down, they should have supplied us with a suspender belt. In spite of my pleas none of the female staff on the ward would lend me any. I used to go round with the tea trolley and wash up in the kitchen with the damn things hanging round my knees; I was forever hitching them up, much to the amusement of the nurses.

After four weeks I was again ready for home and to become an out-patient again, this time at the blood clinic. The procedure there was quite simple really, it was just a pinprick in the thumb and the collecting of a little blood which was put into a clotting machine. The length of time it took to clot was the guide that the doctor used to prescribe your Warfarin tablets. Sometimes you had to go weekly, monthly or even longer. This clinic was by far the largest out-patients' clinic I ever attended regularly, with an average of 70 patients. It needed to be well organised or it became a shambles with people milling everywhere in utter chaos, with patients glaring at each other and complaining to the overworked nurse.

25

Four years went by with only the periodical visit to physiotherapy for treatment to my left leg or my back. Pain in the
leg was constant, with the level of pain being bad or bloody
awful, never anything better than bad, but by now I had
learned to live with it. Pain at some level or other had been
with me since 1961 and it was now 1985.

It was this year that I had something completely new,
bladder trouble. I could remember back to 1964 when I was
in a surgical ward (just temporarily) after one of my operations, and then I thought that they were all poorly middle
aged men, and now here I was, one of them. A 57 year old
man with a bladder that didn't work as it should. It was
very inconsistent and didn't even empty as it should. I was
a cross between a desert camel and a seven months pregnant woman.

It was soon cleared up once they had me in the hospital;
it took only a small prostrate operation when they stretched
the neck of the bladder. I was glad I was asleep at the time.
When I awoke I was the possessor of a 'urine handbag', to
which I was attached by a long length of rubber tubing that
went up my penis to my bladder, it was a catheter. I had
often been threatened with one in the past but now here I
was in bed with my own external water works. Not a pretty
sight! In reality it wasn't as bad as I had often thought in
the past. The most important rule being not to forget your
'handbag' when you went a walkabout, the result of that
could be disastrous as the bag tube came away from the
catheter and you finished up with wet legs or even a very
wet bed.

It was whilst I was there that they discovered another possible reason for some of my persistent backache, and that was that I had a pair of calcified kidneys. I wasn't bothered overmuch, for in spite of the condition they both worked well enough, and as far as I knew they would continue to do so.

After a few days my catheter was removed with a resounding 'plop' similar to the uncorking of a wine bottle. To prevent the possibility of thrombosis I was back on Hefrin again with the usual stomach injections and repeated blood tests until they were at last satisfied, and I could go home again and become, once more, an out-patient.

26

1986 was not a good year for me; it started badly and slowly deteriorated as the weeks went by. I was working too hard and under lots of pressures. When I came home in the evenings I was utterly exhausted but I loved the work, and all of my colleagues were super caring people, but I had been working flat out for over three years. It was a job I would have enjoyed if I was 20 years younger but, alas, I wasn't so the work took its toll.

It was Friday 19 July and I had come home drained, I had nothing left to give. I went to bed early for, with the tiredness, I also didn't feel very well, it was nothing specific other than being completely worn out. I awoke in the early hours feeling very ill and wanting to be sick. I stumbled to the bathroom and started to vomit down the toilet. The next thing I knew was that I was on the floor with my wife kneeling by my side caring for me. She was cleaning me up and putting me in some clean pyjamas. I hadn't remembered falling and as I now had a bad headache we both thought I was having a repeat of the sort of migraine I used to suffer from in my 30s.

Irene put me to bed in the room nearest the bathroom (both sons were away at the time) just in case it happened again. She proved to be very wise indeed, for soon she heard another big bang as I crashed to the bathroom floor again, but this time it was much worse for I was choking on my own vomit. She forced my mouth open and then with her fingers she cleared the vomit from my mouth and throat. I came round as she was cleaning me up again. I wouldn't let her send for the doctor because I was sure it was only migraine, so for the second time she put me back to bed after having changed my pyjamas yet again. I thought that this must be the end of the problem for by now there must have been nothing left for me to be sick with. How wrong I was. Yet another big bang followed as I fell for the third time, but this time as well as swallowing my vomit, I was now nearly swallowing my tongue. Irene had to force my mouth open and clear the vomit again, and also hold my tongue. It was her reactions at that moment that saved my life. She sat in the bathroom beside me until I was feeling well enough to get back to bed, and this time she sent for the doctor.

By this time I felt dreadful, headache, chest pains, and still feeling very sick. The doctor didn't keep us waiting long. He listened to my wife telling him about the night's events. He checked my blood pressure and heart then asked about the chest pain. I just thought that it had been bruised by my falling in the bathroom, or from the constant heaving. It didn't take him long to make up his mind, I needed to be in hospital, and pretty damned quick. My heartbeat was very irregular and my blood pressure was very low. He wasn't sure if I had had a heart attack but he was far from happy with my condition and he wanted me away as soon as possible. In this he was very successful for the ambulance was with us in just under 30 minutes. When they arrived I was sick yet again, but with that out of the way they were able to give me oxygen to help my breathing, for this was deteriorating by the minute.

We arrived at Stepping Hill's A4 ward and I was no sooner transferred to one of the beds than I was back on oxygen. A young nurse then took my blood pressure and what the figures were I don't know, but she almost ran out of the ward. She didn't return, but a staff nurse and a doctor did. They checked my blood pressure again and then it was all systems go. They gave me an ECG, the staff nurse did a dry shave on my chest with apologies, then fastened me to a heart monitor. My heart was racing but my blood pressure was dangerously low. The doctor then put a needle into the back of my hand and fastened a drip to it. By this time I was critically ill so everything was being done at a rapid rate and everyone seemed to care. In the middle of all this activity I was still being sick and that wasn't helping them at all.

When at last they had completed everything there was to do – the monitor, the drip and the oxygen – they prepared to leave me to just one watchful nurse. But before he went, the doctor injected a hypodermic needle into my drip monitor, and as he did so he said, 'This will make you sleep, it is heroin, so don't make a habit of it!' I smiled and thanked him, but behind the oxygen mask they could not see or hear either.

The nurse pulled back the curtains and brought in my wife and friends. My wife later told me that when she saw me she told herself that she wouldn't be taking me home this time. I didn't blame her for I felt, and must have looked, terrible. The heroin soon did its task and I was asleep in no time. How long I slept I had no idea, but when I woke I was still feeling awful, and to make matters worse I was sick again. Fortunately, an attentive nurse was by my side at once with a receiver and a caring word, and when I had finished she wiped my head and face with a cool cloth.

It was the x-ray people who came to see me next, and after putting the plate behind my back, they took just the one picture they required. This was the beginning of a busy spell; it was blood pressure, pulse and temperature by the nurses, then another injection by the doctor. Another doctor who wanted some blood quickly followed this, but this time it was simple and painless. After all this activity I went back to sleep.

I got a shock the next time I woke, for it was dark with only very dim night lights except for one light where the two night nurses sat, one reading and one knitting. As I moved to ease my aching back they must have seen or heard me for they both came over to check that I was alright, and to enquire whether I had any chest pain. I told them that I didn't feel too bad but that I was very thirsty.

189

They asked me how I would like a cup of tea, and I was eager to accept with thanks. I was told to lie as still as possible and my tea came in a beaker. I didn't mind, it saved me worrying about spilling it on the sheets. All I hoped was that once the tea was down, it would stay down. Unfortunately it didn't, and I soon had my head in a receiver.

After this I was wide-awake, and as it was the early hours I watched the daylight come, the arrival of the 6 a.m. reveille, and the nurses to their action stations. As for me, it was blood pressure, pulse and temperature, and my drip bag changed, and then I was given a quick wash, but no shave. I offered to shave myself but was refused point blank, because, they explained, I was on strict bed rest. Breakfast came and went, but I wasn't interested for food was the last thing that I needed, and after my beaker of tea in the night and its consequences, I wasn't bothered with a drink either.

It was now Sunday morning. I just couldn't believe it for so much seemed to have happened since I went to bed on Friday night. My thoughts were interrupted by the arrival of Sister and the doctor. Everything was checked again and some more blood taken. They then both emphasised how lucky I had been, and that I was to have complete rest for about ten days, and also that I was to keep talking down to a minimum with both nurses and patients. Now the rest I could help them with, for I would do as I had been told, but my tongue worked like a metronome, it was hardly ever still. I didn't know it then, but my voice and I were heading for trouble with a capital 'T'.

Sunday is normally a quiet day on the wards so I was able to get plenty of sleep and rest. I wasn't interested in the papers, which was strange for me, and I didn't want to break the rules by chatting to my neighbours. Anyway, all it was so far was smiles and quiet introductions. My wife was a little happier when she saw me in the afternoon, for at least I looked slightly better than I had on the fateful

Saturday morning. Not a lot, but there was a little improvement.

One of the first jobs on Monday morning was to measure me for another pair of white anti-thrombosis stockings. After that there were more injections, and later in the morning came the ladies from the pathology department with their little cards, hunting for victims. I had got to know them well over my years in this hospital, and with the type of blood I had, I always seemed to be first on their list. It was either a thumb prick or a full syringe job, and their trolleys looked like a day out in Sainsbury's butcher's department. It was surprising just how gentle some of the ladies were, and then there were the odd few that were the exact opposite and would have been more suited to working in a joiner's shop.

The day was quiet, and about now my jaw was aching to work, I wanted to talk to someone. Fortunately, there was a guy called George from Buxton. Now, he wasn't on bed rest and wandered aimlessly about or curled up on his bed and tried to sleep the day away. He came over to talk to me when Sister was out of the ward. It appeared that he was waiting to go the MRI for a bypass operation, he had been waiting for a few weeks and he was very bored with life. We hit it off immediately, and through him I was able to converse with the chap in the next bed to my right. He was called Harry and he was also to lie very quietly for he had recently suffered a bad heart attack, and he was in his 70s. It didn't take long to realise that we all had the same kind of humour, and the same 'gift of the gab', so with George as the go-between we were soon exchanging jokes and experiences and laughing out loud. The nurses told us to be quiet or they would have to tell Sister, so we broke up the party for a while and lay still and quiet. It was not long after this that I had my first chest pains since the fateful night, they weren't very bad but they were there so I mentioned it to one of the nurses. Off she went to come back with some tablets for under my tongue, and I was again cautioned about too much talking. Harry also had

191

pain himself and required tablets, only George got off scot-free so it proved that they knew what they were talking about when they warned us all to be quiet and rest.

Now the person on my left-hand side, well he was a pain, to the nurses, Doctors and everyone concerned with him. He complained about the bed, the food and the staff, no matter who it was. He was constantly complaining about his supposedly bad back, he went on for hours on end. He waylaid every available person about his troubles and was an out and out bore, but strangely he never mentioned his heart, and he had a bad enough one. I had to listen to his endless moans all day, but when he turned to me to start, I would pretend to be asleep rather than fall out with him, which would do us both no good.

On the Wednesday I came off my monitor, I still had the drip but it was a good step forward. Also, my new white stockings arrived, and they caused some disturbance for the nurse who had to help me put them on. Like the others they covered the whole of the leg from thigh to toes, and as she lifted each leg in turn, there were whistles and catcalls from the rest of the ward. Without the wires from my chest to my monitor I suddenly found that I had much more freedom to lean over and chat to Harry and George. The subjects were endless; it was football, cricket, politics, hospitals and doctors. Oh, and the royal wedding day! According to Sister, even those that weren't, had to be royalists for the day. The ward was gaily decorated with pictures of the royal couple on all the walls, and Sister bought sherry and cakes. All of us who were able had to participate in the proceedings and not make any derogatory remarks about the royal couple: if you did, in the earshot of Sister, you were in for trouble. My God, for an Irish Sister she was an out and out royalist. Once the thing started on the distant TV screen you could hear a pin drop for she had that kind of power over us. From my bed, and with my eyesight, my view of the royal occasion was just a blur, but I made my peace with Sister by saying how lovely everyone looked. I was true I know, but I couldn't see it from where I was, tha was for sure. After the actual wedding ceremony itself we all received our small sherry and piece of cake to celebrate, and then the ward was back to normal, its usual hive of industry.

The following morning it was discipline as usual, with the Sister very much in charge of the ward, the nurses, and almost all of the patients. I was feeling better for my drip had been removed and I was going to be allowed to sit out of bed for one hour in the armchair. I couldn't wait; I had even shaved myself as well so this really was a progress day. I felt that if I kept this up I would be home in a couple of days. It was all pie in the sky. Because I was up and in a chair I wrongly assumed that the talking ban was lifted, so my mouth prattled forever on. I chatted to the nurses, to porters, to physiotherapists and to nearby patients. The longer I talked, the more my voice was raised as I conversed with patients on the other side of the ward. Then suddenly, after only half of my allotted time had passed, I didn't feel at all well. There were pains in my chest and I felt dreadfully weak, so I quietly asked a passing nurse if I could go back to bed. She told me to sit quietly and not to move, and off she went, to return with Sister. She looked at me sternly.

'Have you much pain?' she asked me sharply.

'I have Sister, I have truly,' I answered quietly. They drew the curtains around my bed and helped me off with my dressing gown and slippers and got me safely into bed. I felt dreadful! I had the pain in my chest and I was not breathing easily. To help me they gave me oxygen for a few minutes until my breathing was back to normal. Sister gave me two tablets to put under my tongue, then left me for a while, but not for long for she then returned with the doctor. He checked my blood pressure and pulse then listened to my heart. He asked if the tablets had eased the pain at all, and I told him that they hadn't much, so it was decided that I would have to have another injection. As I still had my Venthlon in, this was going to give me no problem, and after the injection he told me to lie back and rest and to speak to no one. It was Sister who put it more bluntly.

193

'I don't want to hear your voice going yakity, yakity, yak to anyone for the rest of the day!' Well she needn't have worried, I was scared, and remembered too well the state I had been in just a few days ago.

For my sins I was put back on bed rest only for the next couple of days. The only freedom was being able to go to the toilet in a chair, pushed or pulled by a nurse. The waterworks were great and functioning perfectly, but the bowels were a different matter. I hadn't been since I was brought in, and that was nearly a week ago, but I felt that I needed to go now so I called for a chair. The nurse soon arrived with the vehicle, and I was on my way. When we eventually got there she helped me the two or three steps from the chair to the loo. It was then that she spelled out the ward rules, definitely no straining or pushing, keep the door open, and stay where I was when I had finished as someone would have to take me back to my bed in a chair. I promised to obey all the rules. Now feeling that you want to perform and the actual act are two very different things, especially when you are not even allowed to strain. In hospitals in the past I had always been able to heave and push until the whole act was a success. This was different, I really wanted to go but couldn't get a start, it was agony. I puffed and panted, but all to no avail, all I did was to exhaust myself and I was glad when the nurse arrived back to see how I was progressing.

'No luck nurse,' I said weakly.

'Never mind, I will mention it to Sister for you,' she said as she wheeled me back to my bed. She helped me out of the chair and onto the bed where I collapsed in a heap. I closed my eyes and was soon asleep, but not for long. I woke to see Sister standing by my bed.

'Why haven't you asked for opening medicine if you are so constipated? I always ask about your bowels!'

In my defence I said, 'Well I haven't felt the need to go to the toilet before, and normally I have no trouble in that direction, no trouble at all.'

'Well being in hospital makes it different, you are not

getting any exercise and you are not eating as much food. I will soon put that right when I come round with the drugs trolley, I will see that you go without straining.' By God she was as good as her word, she gave me a potion from the drugs trolley, together with my other medication.

Hours passed but with no effect, then the night staff arrived and cheerfully went about their duties. They went around making sure that everyone was comfortable for the night, this was sometimes just to put the bed rests down and fluff up your pillows, but there was always the hard side for them. This was when they had to bed down the really sick and helpless patients, mainly the men who had suffered various degrees of strokes, making some of them incapable of doing anything for themselves at all. They had their fair share of these. There were also some patients who had to be turned by the nurses physically, sometimes two or three times a night, and without fail there would be soiled beds to be remade. The duty hours from 9 p.m. were one constant hard grind, and yet nearly always, time allowing, they would supply a bedtime drink.

Some nights when it was the duty ward, there would be patients arriving at all hours. The nurses would then be joined by the duty doctors, both male and female, and these people never seemed to be off duty. Heaven knows when they slept, or if they ever did. They would be dealing with heart attacks, strokes, angina or drugs overdoses. Their tours of duty called for alertness, sincerity and efficiency and a lot of stamina. God knows where they got it from.

With the help of sleeping tablets I usually slept through the night's events unless I myself was in trouble with my angina. This one time I did awake, not with the angina, but with a very urgent call of nature. I called out in a quiet but desperate voice, 'Nurse, I need to go to the loo,' then hastily I added, 'it's urgent please, and no it is not just a bottle I need.' One of the nurses dashed off and returned with a commode.

'Oh nurse, not that! Please wheel me to the loo, it will be

better for everyone, especially you two for I haven't been since I came in.' The staff nurse granted my request.

'Straight there, and the nurse will wait with you, and above all no straining.' Little did she know that the only straining that was happening was me trying to hold things back. They helped me out of bed onto the portable commode, and I was wheeled down to the toilets at a fairly fast pace, with all being done quietly so as not to disturb anyone. When we arrived the nurse helped me to the toilet.

'I will wait outside the door, just call me when you have finished.' I had only just sat down when my bowels started to function for the first time in days. There was no need to strain or push, it simply flew away from me with no effort at all. It felt great but I must have stunk out the whole area for I could hear the nurse opening windows.

'Are you alright now Raymond, can you manage to clean yourself or do you need any help?' She must have been very happy when I said I could manage. I felt exhausted but great.

'Ready, nurse' I said as I opened the door.

'Good God Raymond you needed that. Now do you want to wash your hands?' What a question.

'Yes please,' I whispered as she wheeled me to the wash basin at the top of the ward. A short stay there, then back to bed. I felt great.

Later that day I was told that I was now allowed to go to the bathroom and toilet on my own. Now this really was progress. Other than that I had to sit in my chair by my bed and not go round the ward talking to all and sundry. The message from Sister was loud and clear, break the rules and it was back to bed rest.

My neighbour was still confined to his bed, but we could converse quietly without upsetting anyone. George used to come across and join us as soon as Sister was off duty. We swapped many a good story about our past experiences in hospitals. It certainly helped the hours go by. By this time was beginning to feel so much better that it was becoming obvious that with luck I could be going home soon. All th tests showed no heart attack, but heart failure, and that I now suffered from angina. So that was something on the bright side: no heart attack.

The following morning at washing time, all the curtains were drawn around the patients who were bed bound. Harry was one of these, so George and I slipped unseen behind his curtains and plonked ourselves, one either side of him in bed.

A voice called out, 'Have you finished Harry?' We looked at each other in panic for it was Sister herself.

'Yes Sister, I have finished.' With a flourish the curtains were opened, to reveal all three of us in the same bed. It was like the three men in a boat. She was speechless, her face a picture of horror and confusion. But only at first, because before she could chastise us the whole ward burst into laughter, patients and nurses alike, so she herself saw the funny side of it, and thankfully her only remarks were 'You three are like children!' Then she left the ward, bound for her office where we believe she burst into laughter.

My young doctor told me that I might be allowed home on Saturday. They had stopped pumping needles of Hefrin into my stomach, and they had also removed my Ventflon from my hand. The pathology laboratory ladies had taken my last armful of blood so that they could sort out my Warfarin dosage. Things were looking good. Friday was the consultant's round day, and also the day for decisions, out or not out. Now the ward practice was to draw just the bed dividing curtains only, so we were all screened off from each other. There was to be no talking, just silence. It was quite understandable really. Suddenly, out of the silence, someone broke wind, it was just one loud and long fart. It echoed around the ward, and instantly and in unison, Harry and I said out loud, 'I'll name that tune in one!' The whole ward cracked up laughing, patients and nurses alike. Fortunately for both of us, the doctors hadn't yet come into the ward, and they weren't ours anyway. So the nurses were quickly trying to restore order before they arrived, but Harry and I were laughing so much that we couldn't stop, and tears were rolling down our cheeks. In a flash, a staff nurse arrived at my bedside with the 'loo' trolley.

'Come on, in you get, Sister's orders!' I wasn't going to argue with that, so I was sat on the seat and rushed to the toilet.

'And here you stay until this ward round is over, and try to compose yourself ready for your own consultant.' Compose myself? It was not going to be easy, I was shaking with uncontrollable laughter, and tears were still running down my cheeks. I was collected by the same staff nurse fifteen minutes later.

'Now, don't you speak to Harry when you get back or Sister will go barmy. Your doctors are in the office.' I did as I was told and was able to control myself as she wheeled me back to bed. The curtains were still dividing the beds. My doctors arrived accompanied by a stern looking Sister. The doctor who had been looking after me (the consultant had been away on holiday) explained all about my case. Between them they decided that I could go home as soon as my Warfarin dosage was sorted out. Before he finally moved off, the consultant asked, 'How old are you?'

I replied, 'Fifty-eight.'

'I think we will refer you to Wythenshawe,' he said, and left me to ponder on the remark.

Two days later I was discharged with my mixed bag of tablets for medication, together with my red card for the anticoagulant clinic, which told me to report to the pathology laboratory in two days time for another blood test. So here I was, once more an out-patient, for heaven knows how long this time. I had been attending this clinic on and off since 1973, fifteen years in all, so I knew already that at this clinic you had to be a patient out-patient and just wait your turn. On average there were usually between 60 and 70 people attending the clinic at any one time.

27

I had been going along for a regular fortnightly visit for about four months when suddenly I was back in hospital again.

I had not felt well in the afternoon when I was out with friends, but two tablets under my tongue had soon had me feeling better. On my arrival home I decided to have a hot bath to relieve the arthritis in my legs and back before I had my evening meal. It was something that I had done often over the past years but this time it was going to be different.

After my bath as I was drying myself, I felt unwell. I had chest pain and felt quite breathless so I decided to have a rest on the bed, but instead of this helping me I seemed to get worse. I knew I was in trouble again. I banged on the floor to try to attract the attention of my family but no-one heard me, and it was only when my meal was ready and my son called for me, that anyone heard me crying for help. My wife and son responded immediately, for by now my chest pain and breathing were much worse.

This time my wife decided not to wait for a call-out doctor, but to phone 999 and ask for an ambulance at once, for she wasn't sure if it was a heart attack this time. When the ambulance men saw me they told her that she had done the right thing, but because it was a 999 call they would have to take me to Stockport Infirmary's Accident Unit. From there I was transferred by ambulance to Stepping Hill, and into ward A12 (A4 and the Coronary Care Unit were full). The ambulance men lifted me into the bed, and then I waited to be seen by a nurse. To my pleasant surprise the nurse in charge was the one who was the first nurse to see me when I was in A4 the previous July.

'Oh Raymond, not you again!' she said, and then she did my blood pressure and pulse. As I wasn't breathing too well, she put me on oxygen and told me that the doctor would be round to see me soon.

She was as good as her word, for within minutes I had a visit from a young Chinese doctor who examined me for the second time that night, the first time was by the staff at the Infirmary, and he asked me all the usual questions about previous illnesses etc. I think he wished he hadn't bothered. As I still had trouble with my breathing, and also still had some chest pain, he decided to put another Ventflon in my right hand. I didn't mind that because it made having injections later a very simple operation indeed. So firstly it was an injection into the Ventflon, and then the removal of some blood from my left arm for testing. Next was the arrival of a portable x-ray machine, so as usual I was wedged into the right position and had my picture taken. Then followed another ECG test. It was a very busy spell indeed, but soon it was all over and I could lie back and relax, breathing nice and easily with the aid of the oxygen, and before long I drifted off to sleep.

The next thing I knew, I was being asked if I wanted an early morning drink, for it was the start of a new day. I said 'yes please' and as I sat up to drink the tea, I looked about me to see where I was. I found myself in a four-bedded ward. This was a new experience for me, but not one that I was going to enjoy. Unfortunately, the ward consisted of one drugs overdose, one fellow who was very ill and speechless after a stroke, and one very odd guy who derided everyone – nurses, doctors and any other patient who passed his bed. It was the doctors though who were his main target, especially the Asian or Chinese doctors. He was very insulting, but all the medical staff were very tolerant, God knows how, or why. As soon as he saw me in the opposite corner I was straight to the top of his hate list perhaps he thought my 'Menorcan' tan made me look like one of his racist targets. The Sister told me that for some strange reason it happened to anyone who had the bed I was in. He called me all the names he could think of, then, when he ran out of names, he worked his way through some swear book. He was never short of insults. My only defence, without getting highly involved in a battle of words, was to pretend to be asleep and ignore him. Not easy for me I can assure you.

It wasn't long before Sister decided that my condition would not be improved by the constant tirade of abuse, so she moved me next door into the nine-bedded section of the ward. At about this time I was experiencing lots of chest pain so I was behaving myself by being as quiet as I could.

As it happened, my date for an appointment at Wythenshawe arrived whilst I was in the ward, so it was decided that I should keep it and go from A12 by ambulance, accompanied by a staff nurse. It was a good job she was with me, for I was not very well at all. The staff nurse was quite concerned, and managed to arrange for me to be seen by the cardiologist quickly. I had a chest x-ray and ECG, and then was seen by a doctor who, years before, had arranged for my mother to have a pacemaker. He examined me and decided that I should have an angiogram the following week. So with that we were finished for the day, and that meant that we could go back to Stepping Hill, my nurse and I. It was now almost 11.30 a.m.

She duly returned me to the main hall and reported to the ambulance controller that we were ready to go. Now being ready to go from a Manchester hospital and actually getting to Stepping Hill is indeed another matter. Oh, there are plenty of ambulances plying their trade in the Greater Manchester area, and slowly but surely they were emptying the main hall of out-patients going to Manchester addresses. But for anyone like us, trying to return to Stockport or Cheshire is a horse of a completely different colour, for we had to wait for a Cheshire ambulance to come for us. By this time it was one o'clock and we were both very hungry indeed and extremely cold. That large waiting room at

Wythenshawe was not a place to be on a very cold November day, dressed only in pyjamas and a dressing-gown. I was doing my best to keep warm and only managing it because the nurse had wrapped her cloak around my legs. She was freezing. Every time the door opened it seemed as if the icy wind was coming directly from Siberia.

We hadn't got a penny between us for a drink or a bite to eat, so although there was a large café in the hall, it was no use because we were penniless. My nurse explained our predicament but all they could do, they said, was to let us have two paper cups of tea, but no food. It was well turned two o'clock and it was colder than ever, and by this time every other person in the large waiting room had gone, and even the café was closing. So there we were, so obvious sat there that people, nurses, physios and doctors were pointing to us and checking their watches.

Suddenly, on the stroke of three o'clock, a nursing officer all dressed in grey approached and asked us why we had been waiting so long, it appeared that she had passed us a couple of times in the afternoon. The situation was explained to her, and she was horrified that we had waited for so long with no food. She asked if we would like some sandwiches from the hospital cookhouse and I could have kissed her. So to make things easy we both ordered salad when she gave us a choice and she told us that she would arrange it at once.

So we continued to wait. Would the sandwiches or the ambulance arrive first, we wondered. Then, after about 20 minutes, we saw a lone nurse approaching in the distance. We told each other that it couldn't be for us, for she had no food. We were both wrong. She was for us, and she asked, as there was no salad, which other type of sandwich would we like, ham or cheese? We were dumbfounded. Still, it was no use having a go at a young nurse who was only doing what she had been told, so this time we ordered ham to avoid further complications. As we watched her disappear back along the corridor we wondered if she would get back to us before our transport arrived.

It was just after four o'clock when the outside doors opened, and an ambulance man cried, 'Who's for Stepping Hill?' It was obvious that it could only be us for we were the only ones left in the great hall. We looked at each other, decided to forget the sandwiches and go.

The journey back was uneventful and we arrived back at A12 just after five o'clock, both ravenous and thirsty. I was pleased to see that Sister let the staff nurse finish early, she deserved to. I just wanted to get into bed, have my dinner, which had been saved for me, and then sleep, for it had been a long arduous day and I was absolutely knackered.

The staff nurse had brought back a letter, which informed Sister that I was to be returned to Wythenshawe at 8.30 a.m. on Thursday morning (in two days time), for further investigations. It was going to be a case of 'nil by mouth' after supper on Wednesday. Sister confirmed what I had been told at Wythenshawe, that I was to stay overnight. It appeared that they had apparently brought it forward a few days. Still, the sooner the better, it meant that I had less time to think and worry about it.

I didn't sleep much on Wednesday night, even though I did have a sleeping tablet, which was supposed to help me. So I had my bedside bowl and washed and shaved myself very early, and was finished by 6.30 a.m. The ambulance could come for me anytime now; I was ready for them.

8.30 a.m. came and went, and I was still in A12 and not at Wythenshawe where I should have been. I was still there at 9.30 a.m., then at last they arrived. This time my nurse escort was coming with me, then getting a taxi back to Stepping Hill. I was wheeled out to the empty vehicle and climbed inside with the nurse. We drove fifty yards and then stopped again outside the hospital's main corridor. We had to wait whilst they went to another ward for a second patient. I couldn't believe it, it was now almost ten o'clock and we hadn't even left Stepping Hill. They eventually came back with an old lady, but without a nurse escort. She was also going to Wythenshawe; at least that was some consolation. Finally, we left the hospital at 10.30 a.m., already two hours late.

We arrived at Wythenshawe hospital forty minutes later, and the ambulance drew up at the main entrance. At last, I thought, but it was not to be, we were told to wait in the ambulance whilst they took the old lady to her ward. This took another 20 minutes, so by this time I was three hours late. Then the driver got back in the ambulance and started it up again. The nurse asked, 'Where are we going now?'

'The ward you want is much too far to walk,' the driver answered, and he was right, for it took another ten minutes to drive there, and a further five minutes to get up to the ward.

We were greeted by a worried Sister, who asked the nurse escort,

'Where have you been until now? Mr Hill should have been here at 8.30 a.m. and it is now will past 12 o'clock.' She was not happy. I got my piece in first.

'Don't blame me, Sister, I have been ready since 6.30 a.m. this morning.' Whilst the nurse was explaining all the delays to the Sister I was whisked away into the ward by a staff nurse, and told to take off my dressing gown and pyjamas, and my rings and watch, and to put on the gown that was ready for me. By the time I was changed, she was back with an injection for my arm, and a doctor accompanied her.

He said, 'We have been trying to find you all morning, the phone lines between here and A4 have been burning.'

'I am not in A4 this time, I am in A12,' I replied.

'Well you are here now anyway, so just sign this consent form.' I did so without question, they could have been about to cut off my head for all I knew. He then went on to explain very briefly what was going to happen to me. I didn't take it all in because of the urgency of the thing, the porter was now waiting with a trolley to take me wherever the deed was to be done.

It seemed to be an unending journey; I saw more blurred ceiling lights and went up more endless passages than I ever

204

had on my previous visits to hospital theatres. When we eventually arrived I was pushed firstly into an anteroom where there were two girls waiting for me.

'Where have you been until now? We had almost given you up.' So I explained again the reasons for my late arrival. I wasn't with them long before they shouted out loudly, 'Ready!' and off I went into a much larger room where there seemed to be lots of people. Here, I shunted myself off the trolley onto the table in the middle of the room and waited for it all to happen. The important thing was that all the time, someone was talking to me and putting me at ease, so that I felt relaxed and ready for them.

A doctor shook hands, introduced himself to me and sat down by my right side. He pulled my arm towards him and explained that he was going to make a small incision in my arm, to enable him to feed a probe through my arteries and then up to my heart. If I felt up to it, he said, I could watch the whole procedure on the TV screens that seemed to be all around the room. So, after a local anaesthetic, we were off.

I felt hardly anything at all. As I watched him make the small incision, it felt just as though he had gently touched my arm with his nail, no more than that. All the time I was constantly being reassured that everything was fine, I didn't know whether they were nurses or x-ray girls, but no matter who they were they were very caring and made me feel really at ease. Above their heads to my left, I could see the screens. I stared, fascinated at what was happening, I could feel hardly anything yet the probe could be seen gently making its way along my arteries, although of course there were some that it couldn't get through. I felt no pain or even sickness as the operation went on. Then, there was my heart. Incredible. I was told to lie perfectly still and was also told to expect to feel a sensation as though my body was going to be filled with hot water. Now this sounded familiar for I had travelled this road before at the Medical School in Manchester.

The most noticeable thing then was that suddenly the

205

doctor and I were the only ones left. All the ladies had disappeared from sight behind a screen. I had my 'hot flush', then everyone was back and the whole thing was over. Although I was pleased it was over I wished that I had been more observant. The doctor said, 'Well done, but you have very hypersensitive arteries.' I knew I had heard that before.

I was then whisked the long journey back to the ward, put into bed and told to stay there until the morning, and to keep my head down. They didn't have to tell me twice, and after a cup of tea I dropped off to sleep, for it had been a very long day for me.

Soon after breakfast the next morning I had a visit from a doctor who I recognised, I had seen him with other patients on A4 at Stepping Hill.

'Well Mr Hill, it appears that you have very hypersensitive arteries.' I had also been told this by the doctor who had carried out the angiogram, as he was passing his camera through the arteries, and I had been told the same thing in March 1985 when I had to have an insurance examination for my company. Well, I thought to myself, that must be the problem solved, they can't all be wrong. But I wasn't prepared for the doctor's next words, 'So it looks as though it is a by-pass operation for you.' To say that I was shocked was indeed a great understatement. He told me that they were going to send me back to Stepping Hill later in the day.

Back to A12 for a few days, then things seemed to improve, so I was allowed to go and watch TV in the day room. All of a sudden I felt unwell, no chest pain but really ill. I knew that I was in trouble. Fortunately there was another guy in the room with me so I asked him to get a nurse, or anyone. By that time I was in big trouble. The nurses took me back to my bed in the ward and fortunately one of my doctors was with Sister. As soon as he saw me it was all action. He and the nurses pushed me, in my bed, out of the ward, down the corridor and into Coronary Care. I didn't know it at the time but Sister had contacted my family and asked them to get to the hospital at once. It was a struggle for a couple of days, but yet again I went back to A4. It was getting to be a habit.

After a couple more days I had two visitors from Wythenshawe, a senior heart surgeon and one of his assistants. He said that all he wanted to do was to look at the veins in my legs, and then was interested in my knee scars. His last words to me were that the veins would be fine, and that was that. I heard nothing further from anyone.

A few days later I was discharged once again, and began many months as an out-patient at the anti-coagulant clinic at Stepping Hill. So here I was almost hospital-free, having collected so far, two still painful knees, a bloody awful back and now angina. So that was 1986.

Ten months passed by quite uneventfully, with my local surgery looking after me and with no need to visit any hospitals. This in itself was quite an achievement. Then bingo! Here we go again, October 1987. Chest pain, vomiting blood, then out, 999 ambulance dash, but this time when I came round I was in Macclesfield General Hospital, and once again on a monitor and with a drip. Stupidly, I was not happy to be there, I wanted to be in Stepping Hill and more familiar surroundings.

It took just a few days for things to settle down heart wise and I had my first experience of a barium enema to try to find out where the blood was coming from. I didn't like them and they definitely didn't like me because all I could talk about was how good Stepping Hill was compared to them. This didn't go down too well so everyone was pleased when they discharged me.

A few weeks later, in December 1987, a sudden crash and this time I was completely unconscious. My faithful GP came at once and, I was told, took a battling stance to get me a bed in Stepping Hill. Fortunately he won his battle and an ambulance arrived to take me directly to Coronary Care, still unconscious. 48 hours of wonderful nursing and it was back to A4 to be greeted by Sister.

'Oh no, not you again!' I think though, by now I was inwardly quite frightened, for even though I was out of

Coronary Care, I did not feel at all well, so I did exactly as I was told, and by doing so was discharged two days before Christmas. Again I was back in the hands of my local surgery, but forced to retire from work at the age of 57.

Wonder of wonders, this time the years rolled by, until Easter 1992 to be exact. Then more vomiting, more blood, and another 999 back to Stepping Hill. Plasma and blood transfusions, two pints of each. Gastro enteritis was diagnosed which took twelve days to clear.

I wondered if I had finished with hospitals, it was 1973 when I had first arrived at Stepping Hill (which so nearly could have been the last visit). Twenty-five years, a Silver Jubilee.

28

Eight months later I was back again at the surgery. I was being taken on by a new young doctor who was, and is, first class. I was now decidedly not at my best – bouts of angina, and very down – so he had blood samples taken on an urgent basis. The speed of the results took me completely by surprise, for just two days later my doctor phoned me at home and told me to report to ward A12 as early as possible the following morning – Saturday. It was December 1992.

My loyal friends got me there before 9 o'clock, and even then we hadn't beaten the doctors and staff, for they were there with my bed ready, and more importantly, with five pints of blood at the ready. I was told that my blood count was dangerously low at 5.5, and the transfusion was to be slow, five pints over 48 hours. This was because, as well as everything else, I was now anaemic. Well, I said to myself, this is something completely new.

The cardiologist told me that he was convinced that I must be losing blood from somewhere, so commenced more tests, more tubes and more x-rays, all with no answer to the problem. It was then decided that I would have my second barium x-ray, another tube and all that went with it. The consultant said that he was sorry, but it hadn't provided him with the answer to my blood loss, the only thing actually proven was that I, like half of the adult population, had diverticulitis. There still no answer, though, to the question of where the blood was coming from, or even from where it was escaping.

I had been on the anti-coagulant drug Warfarin on and off since my near early demise in 1973. Twenty-five years, a very long time! The last eleven years had seen me at the anti-coagulant clinic almost every month in that time. The cardiologist, because of the mysterious blood loss, decided to gamble and take me off Warfarin completely. A gamble that, to the present day has worked completely.

Luckily for me, Stepping Hill and its super doctors, and of course my own GP have now, on the whole, with the medication that they have put me on, kept me on an even keel. But for how long, we shall have to wait and see.

The first months of 1993 saw me seriously troubled with severe headaches, especially in my temple areas and often into my jaw regions. Was it my migraines back to haunt me from the 60s? I don't think my GP needed the blood tests to tell him what was wrong, but we waited. Then it was confirmed that what he had thought was correct, temporal arteritis. The blood showed my ESR (Erythrocyte Sedimentation Rate) to be 58 against a normal 20 for someone of my age. Subsequent tests saw the figure rise to 66, 77 then 84. So, on my next six monthly visit to my cardiologist it was decided to do a biopsy of the artery on my left temple. By this time I was on a heavy dose of Predisilone (steroids). So it was back into Stepping Hill, but this time only for one day into their new day care ward. It was only minor surgery with a piece of artery being removed under a local anaesthetic. The results were better than expected, that was something. Steroid treatment continued.

Early in 1994, new pains. God, what now? I had been having more trouble than usual with my left leg and needed more help from the pyhsios attached to our local surgery. The present treatment was with a 'tens' machine, which is supposed to be, in basic simple jargon, the act of an electric current telling your brain that you are not in pain. To me it just seemed to be a masochistic way of giving yourself one pain impulse to forget another. Though me being me, I did as I always did, what I was told. Through all my NHS years, I assumed that they knew best. Apart, of course, from a couple of orthopaedic surgeons from my past.

The severe new pain was my spine and the whole left

side of my back. I had assumed at first that it was just my old bad back giving me much more pain than usual. Lucky me though, I was blessed with a 'physio-terrorist', but with a top class girl who looked at my back and reported her fears to my doctor. Eureka! Another hospital, Stockport Infirmary this time. Their x-ray department showed spinal fractures, but the radiologist looked at the x-ray and just said, 'Are you on steroids Mr Hill?' which didn't mean anything to me at the time. Then in March, a scan at Stepping Hill proved that I now suffered from spinal osteoporosis, complete with fractures. My height was now 5'4" compared to my previous 5'8" three years ago. Perhaps now was the time to seek employment with Snow White.

At about this time something occurred which made me have to think about a new arrival, a small blemish or spot on my left temple, which, no matter which cream I tried from my collection, would not heal up. My wife, Irene, kept telling me to see my GP with it, but I didn't! Soon afterwards I wasn't too well, generally quite run down in fact, so off to the surgery for quick check-up, and she didn't miss the opportunity.

'What about this?' she asked the doctor. He looked, then in only a short time I was seen by a dermatologist, who in turn referred me to Christie's hospital. Now this was new, for this place is an oasis in a sea of cancer sufferers, and we are now talking serious illness and brave people. I certainly felt a fool and a fraud in that company. It turned out to be a small skin cancer, which fortunately, two minutes of radiation cleared. I didn't belong in that place, these people were really ill.

29

It was now March 1995, and on one of my check-ups with my cardiologist at Stepping Hill I was in a lot of pain, seemingly everywhere. He decided that I should see another consultant, this time a rheumatologist. He examined me at Stepping Hill, and, as good as I knew him to be, he just left me very confused. Even though my ESR was a high 68 he said that he wasn't convinced that I had temporal arteritis. He said that although I had all the symptoms, when he had examined me once back in the 1980s (which I couldn't remember), I had all the symptoms then as well. What he could tell me was that I had severe fybro-myalgia, and that was where most of my pain was coming from. To say I was confused was an understatement. I felt like the mushroom that is covered with manure (shit!) and left to its own ends in the dark.

Eight months later, November 1995, and I felt that the poor mushroom had died, My back was unbearable, that high pain threshold I was supposed to have had in the past had died with that bloody mushroom, Back to Stockport Infirmary and an orthopaedic surgeon. Here we go again.

He laid his hands on my back, not too gently, and I nearly went through the roof of the old hospital. He realised his mistake and was immediately sorry. Now, as well as the increase of pain, some painful lumps had appeared on the left side of my back. Again the physiotherapist spotted these. Blood tests, x-rays and a scan at Stepping Hill followed. Two days later my wife and I returned for the results.

'Now, the good news is that the lumps on your back are not what we feared.' As we had also feared the same thing,

212

we were relieved. 'But the bad news is that you have severe spinal osteoporosis with fractures, and your spine is being forced over to the left, causing the great pain.' He then added, 'Also with pain coming from nerve ends.' So this, added to my old back damage from 1973, was not good news to me. He went on, 'There is nothing, as a surgeon, that I can do for you except to refer you to the Pain Clinic at Stepping Hill.'

It took four months to get to the clinic, but in the time I waited there were 16 weeks of acupuncture and 'tens' machine therapy. When was it going to end?

April 1996, and into the day care ward at Stepping Hill – a wonderful place with very caring people. The young Irish pain doctor explained that he was going to try a steroid epidural to relieve the pain, but with no honest promise of success. I couldn't argue with that I supposed, the only thing that confused me was that, to a certain extent, it was steroids which were helping the back anyway. But what was there to lose? So the deed was done and a few hours later, when my legs felt as if they belonged to me again, my son collected me and took me home.

The slight improvement unfortunately lasted only a few days, and after that a ride in any type of vehicle was real pain once more. On reporting this to the pain doctor he decided to try another type of injection, a similar style lumbar puncture, but this time with a heavy dose of anaesthetic and not steroids as before.

The procedure in the day ward was more or less the same, though on this occasion the epidural was to be given by a young lady doctor. All day it had been thundering and lightning with torrential rain, a perfect May day in fact. The lightning flashes seemed to light up the mini theatre we were in, and the rolls of thunder were very, very loud indeed. So, as I bent forward to expose my spine, she was not happy – feeling around for the target, and at the same time jumping with every crash of thunder. She was scared! So, in my way, to ease her fears, I told her not to worry if she missed her mark as I knew where coronary care was, and that I could make my own way there.

'My God,' she said as the needle went in, 'don't joke about things like that.'

A few hours later and I was home again.

Just a few days afterwards the pain was back in earnest, barely nine days this time. When I went back and reported this the doctor decided that epidurals weren't the answer. His firm advice was that as oral morphine gave me no sickness, I must be sure that I took it for my pain and not try to be a hero. And that was that.

30

On one of my periodical out-patient visits, it was decided that I should have another echocardiogram. This I had at Stepping Hill on 15 June 1996.

The results were not of any great importance, a slightly enlarged aorta (who hasn't at my age?) and leaky valves. Strange to say, around now I was going through a bad patch, lots of pain almost everywhere – head, back, legs, bones and muscles. And I was losing weight again, down to almost nine stone. My own surgery, who had looked after me so brilliantly, decided to send me to the Alexandra Hospital in Cheadle, this was also in June. It was, I was told, mainly for an echogram and scan. I met the doctor, who told me what he was going to do, which I knew anyway. The scan went ahead. Liver fine, pancreas fine then calcified kidneys, which we knew about. Then he started to examine my head and began asking many questions about my temporal arteritis, the latest ESR was still 77. When I had answered all of his questions he sat back and told me that my head was waiting to 'explode', and that at my age I should be on 100 milligrams of steroids a day. To be honest I didn't think that I had heard him correctly, so I didn't question it, I just got out, and quickly. It has to be said here that this was my first time in a private sector hospital and it was first class, but all my experiences in National Health hospitals have been equally as good.

I went back to my surgery and my GP, poor lad, was in turmoil. What was he going to do with me – had I got temporal arteritis or not? Even in my own surgery I knew of one doctor who was sure I had. In desperation I think,

215

he arranged for me to see another rheumatologist at another hospital, Macclesfield General.

Before I got there though, I had to wear a 24 hour heart monitor; this was for Stepping Hill. The results weren't bad, it appeared that I had been listening to too many Victor Sylvester dance records for my heart rhythm was 'slow, slow, quick, quick, slow'. No problem to me this, for it was still going.

I eventually got to Macclesfield in September 1996. It was a lady consultant and I was immediately very impressed. Her doctor to patient rapport was brilliant. Her first question was to ask me why I was wearing sunglasses. I was sorry I told her, but sunlight and any bright lights hurt my eyes. Her next question staggered me.

'What are you most afraid of Mr Hill?' That was easy.

'Not death. But I am seriously afraid of having a stroke and being a burden to my wife.' She knew at once that I was sincere.

'Reading through your records you should be dead by now,' she said. She then had me taken into another room by a nurse, who helped me undress. The doctor came in and started to examine me. Feet first. 'Brilliant for your age,' she said, and started to work her way up, asking questions as she came to all my surgical scars. 'Things are starting to deteriorate,' she said, 'and in some cases there is not much left.' She then checked my heart, I told her about the recent ECG and the results. Her reply was that she didn't need an ECG to tell her that. At last she got to my head, eyes, ears and nose (not a pretty sight). As she carefully examined my left eye she said that it was no wonder that I didn't like bright lights as I had a cataract. That was surprising news indeed, for it was less than 12 months since my last eye test. Lastly, it was questions all about my temporal arteritis, headaches and jaw aches. My most recent ESR I told her, was 77. This, she told me, she already knew.

I was then weighed, 9st 2lbs; and measured, 5'3". To think that I used to be 11st 7lbs and 5'8"! Then I got dressed again and went back to her office. She told me that she was going to have me thoroughly checked over, and she was as good as her word. Over a fairly long period of time I had a brain scan, another echocardiogram, a CAT scan, a bone scan, and finally, an x-ray of the point where my left collar bone meets my sternum, for a minor problem. After all of these, I had enough power in me to light up the hospital for a week.

A long time ago I had been furious with my wife for letting a 999 ambulance take me to Macclesfield instead of Stepping Hill, but now I had nothing but praise for them and their efficiency. What a well-organised outfit.

All the scans proved that there was nothing other than osteoporosis (and its fractures), osteo-malacia, and fybro-myalgia causing all the pain. When we started to discuss my temporal arteritis, her opinion seemed to be the same as her counterpart at Stepping Hill, I had every symptom, headaches, jaw ache and a very high ESR, but she didn't think that I did have it. The fybro-myalgia was very bad and that could affect the same areas. Her decision though, was that I would have to stay on steroids permanently.

On the whole, I respected all of the doctors' diagnoses but with the temporal arteritis I was more than somewhat confused.

31

Over the years, hospital life has been like a carousel – in time you always seem to finish at the same place. Now was one of those times: back to the Manchester Royal Infirmary. My cardiologist at Stepping Hill, in his wisdom, decided to send me there to try to find out some answers to the irregular heart beat, headaches, sickness, and on some occasions, fainting or blackouts.

So here we were, in January 1997, walking through the much-changed portals of the Manchester Royal Infirmary. As I joined the throngs of other patients I felt that I could either be in Delhi or Durban, it was much more cosmopolitan than it had been in the mid-1960s and early 1970s. My letter had told me that I was going for a 'tilt table' test, and what that entailed I had absolutely no idea. When my wife and I had first met the doctor a few days earlier, he was another one who took a long time to read through my medical history, he looked at me then said to my wife, 'You do realise that he should be dead,' and then to me, 'but you are not, so let us see what we can do to help you.'

So here I was in the cardiology day ward, Ward 16. Thinking back to day ward treatment at Stepping Hill I thought that this would be the same, a few hours and home. Oh brother, how wrong can you be?

The doctor led me quickly into a partly darkened room; I undressed with the help of a nurse, and lay on his table. So far so good. My man then proceeded to stick electrodes all over me and finally, he wrapped a blood pressure kit on my right arm. He explained what he was going to do to me. When the machine was activated, he would slowly tilt the table until I was in an upright position. The nurse then strapped me Frankenstein-style to the table. I asked him what he hoped to achieve and was stunned when he told me that he hoped that I would black out. He then looked down at me and told me that as this was all to do with heart and blood pressure, he would leave for ten minutes for me to relax and compose myself. What a joke that was going to be.

He came back into the room.

'OK,' he said, 'let us get cracking and get this over with for you.' He sat at his electrical piece of equipment and flicked a switch. Nothing. He switched it off. Then on again and off, but quicker this time. There was Middle-Eastern swearing under his breath. As we both looked at each other we knew that this was not our day.

'Let us try once more,' he said, and flew out of the room in a rush. I could hear him blowing his top outside, Maine Road terrace language. When he returned, very crestfallen, he said, 'What can I say?' I think he was half expecting an explosion from me.

'How about, please come back next week?' was my reply. He then went on to explain that the equipment was over ten years old, and that he hoped that they had some spare parts for it.

'I will ring you as soon as it is repaired.' Personally I wasn't too concerned for myself, more for my good friends who were doing a round trip of 40 miles for nothing. The only thing that really did make me furious was that here we were, in one of the best teaching hospitals in the country, and obviously there were others the same all over the rest of the country, with crap machinery. Yet we were spending millions of pounds on a bloody Millennium Dome that 80 per cent of the country's population didn't want. What a bloody cock-up.

As promised, I was back the following week. This time things went along brilliantly – everything worked, so off we went. Slowly the table began to come into an upright position, and all the time I could feel the pressure of the strapping on my arm inflating and deflating. My teeth were clenched firmly, for I had quite bad pain through the tightness of the chest, then suddenly, I knew I was going to faint.

'That's enough!' he cried, and stopped the whole operation. I was untangled, de-wired, and helped to dress. He went away and came back with a drink for me. He told me that I had low blood pressure and an unsteady heartbeat, and to be very careful with sudden standing and moving, and to watch out for being unsteady.

'Drink plenty of water, use lots of salt, and no alcohol.' Then he told me that he would write to Stepping Hill with his findings. As I made my way home, I wondered to myself whether that would be the last of the MRI.

The following week I had to make a short visit to Macclesfield to see an eye specialist. He confirmed that I would need an operation as soon as my name reached the top of the list in around twelve months or so.

A few weeks went by, hospital-less as both an in- and out-patient, until April 1997. I then went to Stepping Hill for the results from the MRI. It was something completely new to anything else that I had suffered in the past. I was told that my tenth cranial nerve, known as the vagus nerve, had apparently taken it upon itself not to work, which can cause headaches, irregular heartbeat, sickness, being completely unbalanced, and even blackouts. When this was happening, it was a case of taking things very steady, no rushing about and being careful not to stand and immediately move off. It was a matter of learning to drive again, moving through the gears slowly.

The following month it was back to Macclesfield, for even though I had a fantastic appetite, my weight was still a problem. So it was another barium enema. Over the years, hospital nurses and others seemed to have taken great pleasure from sticking tubes up my backside, either to put something in or take something out. On this occasion, the x-ray told them nothing that they didn't already know.

32

On good advice from my own GP and both hospital doctors, my holidays to Menorca had been replaced by short flights to Jersey, and an English hospital just in case. Once again, National Health hospitals and doctors were proved correct.

My poor wife's nights were constantly disturbed by really bad bouts of coughing, which, as usual, caused much pain to my back and ribs (cracked ribs that I had suffered before). So, off to the emergency clinic at Jersey General Hospital in St Helier. No praise can be too great. In less than an hour I had been examined by an Indian doctor who looked at the fluid in my legs, sounded my chest, and then had me x-rayed. The result proved that I had a build-up of fluid in my lungs, not, at the moment, at a serious level, but enough to mean an increase in moduretics, which could lead to more unsteadiness, so to take care. As he said, unfortunately life was a catch 22 situation for me.

Shortly after my return from my holiday, there arrived an invitation from Macclesfield to join one of their doctors (a new name to me) as a guest in their day care unit. What now? I had been told to starve myself from the previous night, and I was to have an endoscopy and flexible sigmoid-oscopy examination. This sounded, to me at least, like something that I had not suffered before.

The doctor came to see me and explained the procedure to me. I realised that I had previously had something similar at either end, but never both at the same time.

'You won't feel a thing, you will be asleep,' I was told. That was a relief indeed. Apart from a polyp, the results were all clear.

221

33

Fourteen months went by with, apart from my out-patient check-ups at Stepping Hill, me being almost hospital free. Then I received a phone call at home from the Manchester Royal Infirmary; it was from the cardiology day care unit once again. I was told that there was a letter in the post, but the call was to ensure that I presented myself the following Friday, with nothing to eat or drink from six o'clock in the morning.

'For what?' I asked. The caller told me that I was to be fitted with a loop recorder. The phone went down, leaving me completely in the dark.

My wife and I arrived at the unit to be greeted by my old 'tilt table' doctor, the Manchester City fan (with his obvious intelligence you would think he would know better).

'Oh no, not you again,' was his greeting.

'Charming! But remember, you sent for me.'

'Off with your top clothes and follow me.' I quickly did this, and in no time at all I was lying on a bed stripped for action. Although I was the patient, he looked awful, black rings under his eyes and unshaven.

'It is pretty obvious that you were out on the town last night.'

His female assistant gave a wry smile.

'Oh no I wasn't,' he said, 'I have a three week old baby girl who hasn't yet realised that she is supposed to sleep at night.' I couldn't resist it.

'My eldest son didn't sleep a night through until he was seven years old!'

'Oh God no!' he groaned. But then it was back to

222

business. 'Do you know why we are fitting you with a loop recorder?' As I didn't even know what it was, I had to say that I had no idea why.

'We, and Stepping Hill think that your heart is slowing down, and the machine that we are going to implant in your chest is like a miniature ECG machine which you will be able to activate with an electric controller.' Oh the wonders of modern science! He told me that before I went through to surgery, he had some tests to do, so I was wired up to another machine. Let's hope this one works, I thought. He said that he was going to have to give me an injection which would make me feel very sick, and would be unpleasant. It can't be that bad, I thought to myself. How wrong I was.

'Bloody hell, it's just like a small angiogram that.' It took me all my time to stop myself from being sick all over him.

'That's it for now.' He explained that, as there were four of us, it would take time but they would be as quick as they could. So back to my bed I went, to wait.

An hour went past, then another and not one of the four of us had moved from our bedsides. Then a poor theatre nurse arrived to tell us that there had been a fault with the sterilisation unit and the operations were off for today. Closely behind her followed our 'doc' clad in green.

'Sorry lads, can't be helped.' Poor doctor.

'What a balls up. Does the Manchester City board run this place as well?' We were all told that we would have to return the following week. What a waste of money that bloody Dome is going to be. Just think what it could be used for in NHS hospitals, and what refurbishment could be achieved.

As good as his word, we were all back the following week, hoping for better luck this time. There was to be no need for a repeat of the injections, much to our relief. The only delay was that there were two angiograms before us, but in no time at all, they were back with us on the ward. One was wheeled, on the theatre trolley, to the bed opposite me. He was told to lie head down, and very still for two hours. I must have one of those faces for the nurse turned

223

to me and explained that the gentleman had had an angiogram and needed rest.

'Don't worry nurse, I won't disturb him. I've been there, seen it all, and got the T-shirt.' This brought a half-smile to her face.

Then, wonder of wonders, I was to be first on the list. Always a good thing I think, to get in there first when everyone is fresh and alert, than to be last and hear the greeting of 'oh not another one!'. There was no trolley ride, just a short walk accompanied by a nurse who was big enough to carry one of us under each arm, but very thoughtful and kind with reassuring words all the way there.

As she took me through the doors into the theatre, I was greeted by, 'Meet Mr Raymond Hill, trouble with a capital T.' Today the doctor was clean-shaven and bright-eyed.

The theatre nurses prepared me with a dry shave on my left chest, and then liberally painted me yellow. Then lastly, the 'doc' gave me my local anaesthetic. After that they all stood about to have a chat about everyone and everything that went on in the hospital. The music that played in the background was too modern for my taste.

'Have we no Bee Gees or Motown?' I asked, but was told that the music wasn't for my benefit, but theirs.

'Are we ready then?' Off we go.

I lay there with my eyes tightly closed to keep out the bright lights. As I had already been lying on my back on the hard table longer than I would have liked, I was not very comfortable. As he made his incision he said, 'Oh no, what a bleeder you are.' I told him that I was often called that, and to be thankful I was not still on Warfarin.

'Now Raymond, this is where it starts to hurt.' This, as he seemed to push and shove away at my chest. Suddenly his bleeper started! 'Sorry, I won't be a minute,' he said.

When he returned quite quickly I said, 'Was that call to tell you to turn to the next page of the manual and carry on from there?' He got his own back by pushing even harder.

A few minutes later he said, 'Well that's that, now for some neat sewing.'

It was then that I said to him, 'I hope you have done a first class job so far.'

'Why is that?' he asked.

'Well, if I pop my clogs next week, someone in the medical school could be looking at your handiwork.'

'That's it, put me under pressure won't you.' To his colleagues he explained that I had recently bequeathed my body to the University. A statement which, from the 'ohs' and 'ahs', was received with a mixed reaction.

'That's it, take him away.' So into a wheelchair I went, back the short journey to the day ward. As I had had enough lying down for the last hour I sat by my bed. My theatre nurse, before she left, advised me to keep my arm as still as possible, which would hopefully, she told me, lessen the bruising. If ever there was an understatement that was it, for within hours the bruising was to show, and the following morning I looked as though I had been kicked in the chest by a horse.

Before that I had a visit from a pleasant plump lady with a large portable ECG machine. She sat on the bed and explained in detail what the loop recorder was for, and how to work it. She gave me a type of 'beam me up Scotty!' gadget, and showed me how to activate the recorder with it. In effect, she told me, it was my own individual ECG machine which I was to use only if I thought I was going to have one of my unusual spells, i.e. fainting or worse. Consequently I had to tell my poor wife what she was telling me. Once activated, the recorder would work for a six minute cycle, and it could do this three times. It was a case then of returning to the MRI ECG unit where they could play my tape on their machine. Indeed it was a really super gadget, and up to now it has only been needed twice.

34

The present situation is this, as far as I know. The skin cancer appears to be back, they could be wrong but they are working on it. The cataract operation on the left eye is due, I hope, early next year as the vision out of it is now practically nil. With the calcified kidneys, I am told that they don't function properly but should last me out. How long is 'out' I wonder? Is 'out' the next day? Is 'out' next week? Is 'out' next month? Is 'out' next year? Or is 'out' yet another decade, when some other doctor or hospital will tell me 'You should have been dead years ago'? Only time will tell. As regards everything else, in the words of one of my hospital doctors, there are very many things wrong with me, but at the moment nothing is life threatening, providing I keep taking all my medication.

So how do you end a book like this? (That is if anyone has read this far.) It would help, before I do that, to tell you why I started it in the first place. Well, it was now, believe it or not, three decades ago!

My wife Irene and I have two doctor friends, one a pathologist at the Manchester University Medical School, the other a Medical Officer of Health for a very large area near Manchester (of course in the length of time it has taken me to finish the book, they are both long since retired). Well I used to sit and tell these friends of the many amusing experiences, and of course, those that were more traumatic, in the numerous hospitals I had been in. So I started, at their insistence, to put it into words as best I could. Fortunately I have a first class memory. Now, if I had finished it as quickly as I had talked about it, then all it

226

would have consisted of would have been hernias, knees, and one or two other bits and pieces, for at that time I was just turned 40. So if you have read it thoroughly, you will know that it has rolled on until I am now 70. Another 30 years of, I hope, not too much boring reading.

How do I end it then?

A few months ago, as I sat waiting in my surgery for my appointment, I picked up an organ donor card. Then, when my number came up, I took it into my GP. He, at first, found it very amusing.

'Raymond, nothing really works.' As usual he was right of course, but I knew I had to give something back to the NHS, and all the hospitals somehow. Then, with the help of a nursing Sister friend, I found the answer.

After talking to my wife and son (who was not too happy at first) I came to my decision. Over the years very many people, both medical and otherwise, never expected me to reach three score years and ten. But I have. This is due only to the love and care of my wife Irene, and of course our magnificent National Health Service and all who work in it. So to find out why and how I have defeated the odds stacked against me and, more importantly, to help future doctors and future patients, I have bequeathed my body to the Manchester University Medical School. This, surely, can only be right.